Cluster headache
mechanisms and management

Lee Kudrow, MD
Director, California Medical Clinic for Headache

Oxford New York Toronto
OXFORD UNIVERSITY PRESS
1980

Oxford University Press, Walton Street, Oxford OX2 6DP

OXFORD LONDON GLASGOW
NEW YORK TORONTO MELBOURNE WELLINGTON
KUALA LUMPUR SINGAPORE JAKARTA HONG KONG TOKYO
DELHI BOMBAY CALCUTTA MADRAS KARACHI
NAIROBI DAR ES SALAAM CAPE TOWN

*Published in the United States by
Oxford University Press, New York*

British Library Cataloguing in Publication Data
Kudrow, Lee
   Cluster headache. – (*Oxford medical
   publications*).
   1. Histamine cephalalgia
   I. Title   II. Series
   616.8'57   RC392   79–41661
   ISBN 0-19-261169-0

*Filmset by Northumberland Press Limited, Gateshead
Printed in Great Britain by
Lowe & Brydone Printers Limited,
Thetford, Norfolk*

Foreword

Donald Dalessio, Chairman, Department of Medicine,
Scripps Clinic, La Jolla, California
Medical science rarely advances by leaps and bounds; in truth, to many patients it must seem as though the advances are measured rather in inches, intermixed with an occasional retreat, the latter not infrequently the handiwork of the health planners. Yet advance it does withal, a tribute to a polyglot group dedicated to new knowledge. Some of this new knowledge is the result of fundamental observations of the basic scientists. Other improvements are technological, for example the diagnostic revolution in neurology engendered by computerized axial tomography of the cranial contents. Yet Pope's dictum still holds, that the proper study of Man is Man, and hence at least a few medical discoveries are still made by alert and careful clinicians, practitioners of medicine, quick of eye and pen, who are able to set down and interpret the vagaries of symptoms their patients describe and cull from them new diagnostic categories which can thereafter be employed by the rest of us.

There is a natural tension between research scientists and clinicians over the subject of clinical research, and this is perhaps a consequence of their different aims and aspirations. Members of research groups consider themselves to be scientists, doing scientific work, and they are probably jealous of the scientific reputation which has been established in the last two decades, often supported in part or in whole by government grants. Some researchers are also physicians (practitioners of medicine, healers), but many have abandoned this role and the active practice of medicine.

In contrast, clinicians do consider themselves as physicians and practitioners, interested in clinical disease states, and in the care of sick and well patients. Some physicians have clinical research interests as well, yet are more likely to be concerned less with disease mechanisms than with clinical trials, or perhaps those disease mechanisms directly related to patient care. To the basic scientist, such research may at times seem trivial, suspect, or lightweight.

Again in contrast, many scientists pursue research and grant support primarily concerned with basic mechanisms of disease or homeostasis; their work is often not aimed at or based upon therapeutic principles. Furthermore, they may not be partially or even slightly interested in disease treatment. In this regard many scientists will feel closer kinship with other non-clinical scientists (biologists and chemists) than they do with clinicians. The clinical researcher must fill the void between bench and bed and it is to him that both scientists and clinicians must turn. It is this person who will encourage research on patients, of an ethical nature, particularly clinical trials, and careful observations of disease states. In a sense, this is goal-oriented clinical research. There is no reason why this activity cannot be of excellent quality, and innovative, though obviously it is limited by the subject matter, since patients talk back, and even occasionally sue.

The situation described above also applies to headache, said to be man's most ubiquitous problem. In the last two decades, and especially in the last ten years, a flood of knowledge about headache has appeared, perhaps in parts related to the proliferation of specialized societies and clinics for the study of this subject. Headache has been inspected, dissected, and teased apart by a variety of clinical researchers from various countries, and gradually the various forms of headache have appeared in a classification to which most physicians can relate. Precision in description has clarified the multiplicity of syndromes sometimes burdened by one or another clinician's names, especially from the past. As John Dirckx observes, eponyms are often tombstone words, and the early descriptions of headache were frequently encumbered by the name of the original descriptor of the syndrome, which produced a bewildering maze of names to be learned, each not signifying much of anything.

This monograph is a welcome change from that tradition. Dr Kudrow has carefully delineated a particular form of headache, cluster headache, and has turned a clear eye on this syndrome as he surveys its aetiology, pathogenesis, frequency, genetics, and treatment. Perhaps the best part of the volume is contained in his own studies and observations of his many patients, ranging from their physical characteristics to the relationships of their headache problems to the vicissitudes of life. In his capacity for observation and detail, Dr Kudrow has set a standard for other clinician observers to follow. His book is a model of clinical research, a small gem, a clear exposition of a clinical problem of significant importance in the population. The material is tightly organized, logical in its sequence, and adequately referenced. The simplicity of his presentation makes for easy understanding by both general physician and specialist alike. It does not answer all of the questions raised regarding this subject; indeed its greatest value may be in the questions it asks and the opportunities thus engendered for subsequent investigations.

Preface

Some years ago, a patient of mine inquired how I had so readily diagnosed his headache condition as cluster headache, when so many other physicians had missed it; I was at a loss to provide him with an acceptable explanation. I was more perplexed with the fact that for the previous ten years the patient had been treated for 'sinus problems', migraine, and dental problems; the latter resulting in root canal procedures and extraction of two innocent teeth.

Unfortunately, such stories are commonly related by patients although with varying circumstances. Paradoxically, cluster headache presents so stereotypically, from patient to patient, and from cluster period to cluster period, as to be considered one of the more easily diagnosable headache disorders.

Since the original and creative scientific endeavours of Harold G. Wolff and his associates, headache disorders, in general, have been gently lifted off the psychiatrist's couch and deposited into the consultation rooms of neurologists and specialists in headache. More recently, organizations such as the American Association for the Study of Headache. World Federation of Neurology, Scandinavian Migraine Society, Italian Migraine Society, and The Migraine Trust in Great Britain have stimulated interest and research throughout the international medical community. As a result, many pathophysiological aspects of headache disorders have been elucidated and have invalidated certain psychological theories relating to chronic and recurring headaches—all to the benefit of the headache sufferer.

Among the various headache disorders, cluster headache has the distinction of being the most painful and, to the discomfort of some patients, the most frequently overlooked diagnosis. This book was prompted by this revelation and in view of the accumulation of information on cluster headache in recent years. Hopefully, it will provide the reader with sufficient clinical material to enable him readily to diagnose cluster headache.

Data on biochemical, hormonal, and vascular changes associated with the cluster attack are presented and form a mosaic of pathophysiological events contributing to cluster headache. Admittedly, pathophysiological voids still exist and some basic questions remain unanswered.

The last chapter of this monograph concerns management of cluster headache patients. Avoidance, symptomatic, and prophylactic treatments are discussed in great detail. Although there is still much to be learned about cluster headache, adequate methods of treatment, as described in this book, are now available to relieve the suffering of the great majority of cluster headache patients.

Encino, California   LK

Acknowledgements

This monograph could not have been written without the interest and cooperation of John R. Graham, MD, Karl Ekbom, MD, James W. Lance, MD, and Ottar Sjaastad, MD.

In addition, I extend my gratitude to E. C. Kunkle, MD, H. Heyck, MD, L. L. Lovshin, MD, M. Anthony, MD, N. T. Mathew, MD, D. Russell, I. Hørven, MD, F. Sakai, MD, and J. S. Meyer, MD, for having shared with me their inner thoughts on the subject of cluster headache.

I am grateful to B. J. Sutkus, PhD for his statistical contributions and to Mr M. H. Mandell for his insatiable interest in the written word. My thanks are also due to Mrs B. Chanin who through her ingenuity with scheduling office hours, enabled me to have the time required to complete this manuscript.

Contents

To my wife, Nedra

1 Classification

Nomenclature and classification

Nomenclature (Table 1.1)

There is virtually no description in the medical literature, prior to 1840, of the syndrome called 'cluster headache'. On that date, Romberg[29] published an account of a headache episode associated with ipsilateral lacrimation, conjunctival redness, and miosis. He believed that this syndrome was due to a tubercular abscess (scrofula) or, curiously enough, to seminal discharge.

In 1867, Möllendorff[27] published an account of a new syndrome which subsequent writers believed was an early description of cluster headache.[6,7,11] It was known as 'red migraine'. It is more likely that Möllendorff described a migraine variant and not cluster headache.

Heyck[17] states that the first accurate description of cluster headache was reported in the German medical literature by Eulenburg in 1878. In his textbook, *Lehrbuch der Nervenkrankheiten*, Eulenburg referred to this disorder as angioparalytic hemicrania.

Table 1.1 Cluster headache—eponyms, misnomers, and other appellations

| Authors | Date | Nomenclature | |
		Eponyms	Other names
Romberg	1840	Description only	
Möllendorff	1867		Red migraine
Eulenburg	1878		Angioparalytic hemicrania
Sluder	1910	Sluder's syndrome	Sphenopalatine neuralgia
			Lower half headache
Bing	1913	Bing's headache	Erythroprosopalgia
		Bing's syndrome	
Harris	1926		Migrainous neuralgia
Harris	1936		Ciliary neuralgia
Vail	1932		Vidian neuralgia
Gardner *et al.*	1947		Greater superficial petrosal neuralgia
Horton *et al.*	1939	Horton's headache	Erythromelalgia
	1952	Horton's syndrome	Histaminic cephalgia
Kunkle *et al.*	1952		Cluster headache

Sluder in 1910[36] and again in 1913[37] described a syndrome often confused with cluster headache. Sphenopalatine ganglion neuralgia, or Sluder's syndrome, is characterized by paroxysms of facial and hemicranial pain followed by spontaneous remissions. However, its sex distribution, quality, duration, and exact location of pain, quite separates it from cluster headache.

The term 'erythroprosopalgia', coined by Bing in 1913[4] is not a commonly used term for cluster headache. The eponym, Bing's headache or Bing's syndrome, is clearly not cluster headache, in the opinion of Ekbom.[8] His objection is based on three characteristics of Bing's syndrome which bear little relationship to cluster:

1. unilateral or *bilateral* distribution of pain.
2. located around the eyes, like a pair of glasses, associated with
3. facial redness and oedema.

An account of cluster headache was published by Wilfred Harris. He referred to this syndrome as 'periodic migrainous neuralgia' in 1926[15] and 'ciliary neuralgia' in 1936.[16] The former term is still commonly used by European clinicians. Harris is to be credited with the first English reporting of this disorder. A critical view of his case histories, however, reveal a mosaic of entities that include cluster headache, atypical facial neuralgia, and migraine. The term 'migrainous neuralgia' is acceptable on the basis of common usage; but it should be recognized as a misnomer, since it is descriptive of neither migraine nor neuralgia.

Attempts to define cluster headache by anatomical nervous pathways are represented by such terms as 'Sluder's sphenopalatine ganglion neuralgia', 'vidian neuralgia', and 'greater superficial petrosal neuralgia'. The selection of these particular nervous pathways is derived from autonomic characteristics and pain distribution of cluster headache. Vail,[38] in 1932, hypothesized that the vidian nerve, formed by the sympathetic deep petrosal and parasympathetic greater superficial petrosal nerves, was the pathway of the cluster headache picture; hence the term 'vidian neuralgia'. Gardner,[12] in 1947, believed that cluster headache was mediated via the greater superficial petrosal nerve and introduced the term 'greater superficial petrosal neuralgia'. Section of this nerve, however, provided excellent results in only 25 per cent of cases. Reportedly,[25] Gardner became somewhat discouraged with these results, and subsequently used this procedure only rarely.

Apparently unaware of previous reports, Horton, MacLean, and Craig[21] in 1939, described 'a new syndrome' and for descriptive purposes, called it 'erythromelalgia of the head'. Their report of 84 patients contains the most accurate description of cluster headache thus far. Since then, Horton[18-20] has published numerous studies of this condition which he later called 'histaminic cephalgia'. In his publication on erythromelalgia, Horton *et al.*[21] first introduced the use of histamine provocation, and from this observation, Horton was to pursue the concept that 'cluster headache' was a histamine-mediated disorder (see Chapter 5).

It was not until 1952 that E. C. Kunkle *et al.*[24] observing the clustering pattern of headache attacks in 30 patients, applied the term 'cluster headache'. It should be noted, however, that K. A. Ekbom[9] had been the first to describe its periodic character quite concisely in 1947.

Following a rather extensive publication on cluster headache by Friedman and Mikropoulos[11] in 1958, the term became generally accepted and formally recognized by the Ad Hoc Committee on Classification of Headache, in 1962[1] and the World Federation of Neurology, Migraine and Research Group in 1969.[39]

Definition. Although cluster headache is classified under vascular headache of the migraine type by the Ad Hoc Committee on Classification of Headache,[1] it is now recognized as an entity distinct and separate from migraine, by many specialists in the field. The chronic type of cluster headache had not been included in this classification. Nor were the following three varieties of cluster headache: cluster-migraine, chronic paroxysmal hemicrania, and cluster-vertigo.

Classification

A modification of the cluster classification is presented here to update and include substantial variants of this disorder (Table 1.2).

Episodic cluster headache is a primary headache disorder. Paroxysms or *attacks* occur in series, interrupted by extended periods of remission. The attacks often occur regularly, at times frequently, throughout the *cluster period*. During this time, susceptibility to headache induction is increased. Headache-free intervals between attacks, occurring within a cluster period, are often called *interim periods*. The majority of patients with cluster headaches have the episodic type.

Table 1.2   Classification of cluster headache

---

1 Episodic (periodic)
2 Chronic
    A Primary
    B Secondary
    C Chronic paroxysmal hemicrania (CPH)
3 Atypical variant
    A Cluster-migraine
    B Cluster-vertigo

Chronic cluster. Rooke, Rushton, and Peters[30] in 1962, noted a chronic pattern among some cluster patients and called it *Horton's headache, chronic type.* It refers to those cases in which remissions do not occur. More specifically, patients having never experienced remissions are considered to be *primary chronic*; whereas those who become chronic, having had episodic patterns, are categorized as *secondary chronic* types. According to Ekbom and Olivarius,[10] chronic cluster headache is distinguished from the episodic type, as follows: absence of a remission period for at least one year, increased attack frequency, and diminished responsiveness to prophylactic drug therapy.

Cluster-migraine, an atypical variant of cluster headache, is described as having components of both disorders. In our experience, these patients may suffer typical migraine headaches in cluster patterns or may exhibit typical cluster symptoms during migraine attacks. Medina and Diamond[26] described seven such cases as an example of the clinical link between migraine and cluster.

Chronic paroxysmal hemicrania was first described by Sjaastad and Dale in 1974.[34] To date, only five patients having this disorder have been reported.[35] It differs from typical chronic cluster in that all known cases are women, attacks are more frequent and shorter in duration, it rarely occurs during sleep hours, and it is dramatically responsive to aspirin or indomethacin.

Cluster-vertigo, a much overlooked, though rare, variant of cluster headache, was first described by Gilbert in 1965.[13] In such cases, episodes of vertigo occur during some or all cluster headache periods, but not during headache remissions. Therefore, the headache and vertigo attacks may share the same mechanism: recurrent paroxysmal multifocal vasodilatation.[13, 14]

Is cluster headache distinct and separate from the migraine syndrome?

The occurrence of cluster and migraine in headaches in the same patient is not mutually exclusive. Approximately 10 per cent of cluster males have migraine headaches periodically, an incidence similar to that of the general male population[22] (see Chapter 5). Because of the 'vascular' nature of cluster headache, it has often been associated with migraine. That is, extracranial vasodilatation is common to both disorders. Since Horton[21] first described cluster headache as a distinct entity, evidence has accumulated which support his contention.

This question is best answered by categorizing clinical, biochemical, and blood-flow data, which when weighed, will support or reject the 'common entity' concept.

Evidence in support of the common entity concept

The clinical resemblance of cluster to migraine headache is limited to unilateral pain occurring in all cases of the former and in approximately 80 per cent of the latter. Also, there has been some question regarding the association of attack onset and REM sleep states. Dexter and Riley[5] reported that migraine and cluster attacks, when occurring in sleep, are associated with REM state. However, a review of their published sleep records reveal that, of nine headache events experienced by three cluster patients during sleep, only three attacks occurred during REM. The remainder occurred in other stages, following REM. In three migraine patients, however, of eight attacks, six occurred during REM. Hence, an association of the cluster attack to the REM state remains questionable.

Extracranial vasodilatation appears to be a common finding in both disorders. Superficial temporal artery enlargement during attacks is associated with pain. Compression of this artery often provides temporary relief. Indeed, Sakai and Meyer[31] have demonstrated increased extracranial blood-flow during attacks in both migraine and cluster patients. They have also demonstrated that cerebral blood-flow increases during cluster and migraine attacks. In the former, however, cerebral blood-flow returns to normal in association with pain relief, but in the latter, persists for as long as one week following pain cessation.[31] In separate Doppler flow studies, decreased blood-flow velocity was recorded from the ipsilateral supraorbital arteries (branch of the internal carotid artery), in both migraine[28] and cluster groups.[23] Hence, cluster and migraine attacks appear to be characterized by similar vascular changes; external carotid artery dilatation and internal carotid artery constriction (Chapter 5).

The two disorders are similar in their response to some symptomatic and prophylactic agents. Migraine and cluster attacks are relieved or prevented by vasoconstrictors, such as ergotamine or methysergide, respectively. Other agents, however, are prophylactically beneficial in one condition but not in the other, as will be discussed later (see Chapter 8).

Patients in both categories share similar personality profiles. This will be discussed in greater detail in Chapter 4.

Evidence against 'common entity' concept (Table 1.3)

As noted earlier, the major clinical feature common to both migraine and cluster attacks is unilateral location of pain. The differences, however, are much greater. Cluster differs from migraine in: periodicity; incidence; familial history incidence; sex distribution; age of onset; attack frequency, duration, and severity; associated symptoms; lack of throbbing components; and behavioural response.

In contrast to migraine, hormonal influences, as observed with menstrual changes and extrinsic oestrogen use, have little effect in cluster headache (see Chapter 3).

The incidence of ulcer disease in cluster populations is significantly greater than among migraineurs (see Chapter 5).

Specific biochemical changes have been associated with each disorder, separately. Platelet serotonin levels were reported to be elevated during the prodromal phase, and decreased in the headache phase of migraine.[2, 33] This change was not found in cluster headache patients[3] (see Chapter 7).

Both conditions respond symptomatically and prophylactically to ergotamine and methysergide, respectively. Propranolol, however, has prophylactic benefit in migraine, but not in cluster headache. Conversely, lithium is a major prophylactic therapeutic agent in cluster headache, but not in migraine. Cluster attacks, unlike those of migraine, are dramatically responsive to oxygen inhalation (Chapter 8). A rationale for the symptomatic benefit of oxygen inhalation in cluster headache has been provided by Sakai and Meyer.[32] In a series of cluster, migraine, and control patients, they

Table 1.3 Differences between cluster and migraine headaches

Characteristics	Headache disorders	
	Cluster	Migraine
Clinical aspects		
General		
Age onset	30 years†	20 years
M : F ratio	> 5 : 1	1 : 3
Incidence	Approx. 1%	M, 10%; F, 22%
+ Medical history	Ulcer history (20%)	None
+ Family history	< 5%	> 50%
Attack profile		
Frequency	1–3 per day†	2 per month
Duration	1 hour†	1 day
Intensity	Excruciating	Severe
Throbbing	Uncommon	Common
Unilat. lacrimation	Common	Uncommon
Unilat. rhinorrhoea	Common	Uncommon
Partial 'Horners'	Common	Uncommon
Behaviour (activity)	Cannot lie still	Must lie still
Hormonal and biochemical changes		
Oestrogen influence	Rare	Common
Plasma serotonin	No change	Increased
Plasma histamine	Increased	No change
CSF acetylcholine	Increased	No change
CBF response to:		
Oxygen (attack-state)	Excessive	Normal
CO_2 (pain-free state)	Normal	Excessive
Medication response to:		
Propranolol	Poor	Excellent
Lithium	Excellent	Poor
Oxygen inhalation	Excellent	Poor

† Average values.

measured cerebral blood-flow responses to oxygen and carbon dioxide, by the ^{133}Xe inhalation method. They found that during cluster attacks, the cerebral vasoconstrictive response to 100 per cent oxygen was excessive. This was not the case in either migraine or control patients. Vasodilatation response to carbon dioxide in migraine subjects, was impaired during the prodrome and headache states, and excessive during the headache-free interval. Although response to carbon dioxide was also impaired during the cluster attack, it was found to be normal during the headache-free interval (Chapter 8).

Considering all evidence, it appears that the major features common to both migraine and cluster headache, are arterial changes. Such changes, however, may be the end result of separate processes. The differences between these disorders are qualitatively significant, and in my opinion, separate each into distinct entities.

References

1 AD HOC COMMITTEE ON CLASSIFICATION OF HEADACHE. *J. Amer. med. Assoc.*, **179**, 717–18 (1962).
2 ANTHONY, M., HINTERBERGER, H., and LANCE, J. W. Plasma serotonin in migraine and stress. *Arch. Neurol. (Chicago)*, **16**, 544–52 (1967).
3 ——, and LANCE, J. W. Histamine and serotonin in cluster headache. *Arch. Neurol.*, **25**, 225–31 (1971).
4 BING, R. *Lehrbuch der Nervenkrankheiten* (1st edn.). Ukban and Schwarzenberg, Berlin (1913).
5 DEXTER, J. D. and RILEY, T. L. Studies in nocturnal migraine. *Headache*, **15**, 51–62 (1975).
6 DUVOISIN, R. E., PARKER, C. W., and KENOYER, W. L. The cluster headache. *Arch. Intern. Med.*, **108**, 111–16 (1961).
7 EADIE, M. J. and SUTHERLAND, J. M. Migrainous neuralgia. *Med. J. Aust.*, **53**, 1053–6 (1966).
8 EKBOM, K. A clinical comparison of cluster headache and migraine. *Acta Neurol. Scand. (Suppl.)*, **4146**, 1–48 (1970).
9 EKBOM, K. A. Ergotamine tartrate orally in Horton's 'histaminic cephalgia' (also called Harris' 'ciliary neuralgia'). *Acta Psychiat. Scand. (Suppl.)*, **46**, 106–13 (1947).
10 EKBOM, K. and OLIVARIUS, B. DE FINE. Chronic migrainous neuralgia— diagnostic and therapeutic aspects. *Headache*, **11**, 97–101 (1971).
11 FRIEDMAN, A. P. and MIKROPOULOS, H. E. Cluster headaches. *Neurology*, **8**, 653–63 (1958).
12 GARDNER, W. J., STOWELL, A., and DUTLINGER, R. Resection of the greater superficial petrosal nerve in the treatment of unilateral headache. *J. Neurosurg.*, **4**, 105–14 (1947).
13 GILBERT, G. J. Meniere's syndrome and cluster headache. Recurrent paroxysmal focal vasodilatation. *J. Amer. med. Assoc.*, **191**, 691–4 (1965).
14 ——. Cluster headache and cluster vertigo. *Headache*, **9**, 195–200 (1970).
15 HARRIS, W. Ciliary (migrainous) neuralgia and its treatment. *Brit. med. J.*, **1**, 457–60 (1936).
16 ——. *Neuritis and neuralgia*. Oxford University Press, London (1926).
17 HEYCK, H. Der Cluster-Kopfschmerz. *Dtsch. med. Wschr.*, **100**, 1292–3 (1975).
18 HORTON, B. T. Histaminic cephalgia. *Lancet*, **72**, 92–8 (1952).
19 ——. Histaminic cephalgia: differential diagnosis and treatment. *Mayo Clin. Proc.*, **31**, 325–33 (1956).
20 ——. Histaminic cephalgia (Horton's headache or syndrome). *Maryland med. J.*, **10**, 178–203 (1961).

21 ——, MacLean, A. R., and Craig, W. M. A new syndrome of vascular headache: results of treatment with histamine: preliminary report. *Mayo Clin. Proc.*, **14**, 257–60 (1939).

22 Kudrow, L. Prevalence of migraine, peptic ulcer, coronary heart disease and hypertension in cluster headache. *Headache*, **16**, 66–9 (1976).

23 ——. Thermographic and Doppler flow asymmetry in cluster headache. *Headache*, **19**, 204–8 (1979).

24 Kunkle, E. C., Pfeiffer, J. B. Jr., Wilhoit, W. M., and Hamrick, L. W. Jr. Recurrent brief headache in 'cluster' pattern. *Trans. Amer. Neurol. Assoc.*, **77**, 240–3 (1952).

25 ——, and Dohn, D. F. Surgical treatment of chronic migrainous neuralgia. *Cleveland Clin. Quart.*, **41**, 189–92 (1974).

26 Medina, J. L. and Diamond, S. The clinical link between migraine and cluster headache. *Arch. Neurol.*, **34**, 470–2 (1977).

27 Möllendorff. Über hemikranie. *Virchow's Arch. Path. Anat.*, **41**, 385–395 (1867).

28 Otis, S. M., Smith, R. A., Kroll, A. D., Krasny, S. E., Seltzer, K. A., and Dalessio, D. J. Vasospasm and vascular headaches: selective vasoconstriction in carotid vascular system measured by the Doppler ophthalmic method in migraineurs. *Headache*, **19**, 200–3 (1979).

29 Romberg, M. H. *A manual of nervous diseases of man* (transl. E. H. Sieveking), London, Syndenham Society (1840).

30 Rooke, E. D., Rushton, J. G., and Peters, G. A. Vasodilating headache: a suggestive classification and results of prophylactic treatment with UML 491 (methysergide). *Proc. Staff Meet. Mayo Clinic*, **37**, 433 (1962).

31 Sakai, F. and Meyer, J. S. Regional cerebral hemodynamics during migraine and cluster headaches measured by the ^{133}Xe inhalation method. *Headache*, **18**, 122–32 (1978).

32 ——, and ——. Abnormal cerebrovascular reactivity in patients with migraine and cluster headache. Presented at the Twentieth Annual Meeting of the American Association for the Study of Headache, Boston (1979).

33 Sicuteri, F. Mast cells and their active substances: the role in the pathogenesis of migraine. *Headache*, **3**, 86–9 (1963).

34 Sjaastad, O. and Dale, I. Evidence for a new (?) treatable headache entity. *Headache*, **14**, 105–8 (1974).

35 ——, Egge, K., Hørven, I., Kayed, K., Lund-Roland, L., Russell, D., and Slørdahl Conradi, I. Chronic paroxysmal hemicrania: mechanical precipitation of attacks. *Headache*, **19**, 31–6 (1979).

36 Sluder, G. Etiology, diagnosis, prognosis and treatment of sphenopalatine ganglion neuralgia. *J. Amer. med. Assoc.*, **61**, 1201–5 (1913).

37 ——. The syndrome of sphenopalatine ganglion neurosis. *Amer. J. med. Sci.*, **140**, 868 (1910).

38 Vail, H. H. Vidian neuralgia. *Ann. Otol. Rhinol. Laryngol.*, **41**, 837 (1932).

39 World Federation of Neurology's Research Group on migraine and headache. *J. neurol. Sci.*, **9**, 202 (1969).

2 Incidence, age of onset, sex, and ethnic distribution

Relative incidence

Ekbom, Ahlborg, and Schele[6] surveyed 9803 eighteen-year-old Swedish males and found a cluster incidence of 0·09 per cent. With the exception of these data, there are no other reports on the prevalence of cluster headache in the general population. In several clinic populations, the incidence of cluster headache, relative to migraine, has been reported. Unfortunately, there appear to be wide discrepancies between these reports. The first such study was reported by Lieder[16] in 1944. Using migraine for a basis for comparison, he found a 13:1 ratio of migraine to cluster headache. Heyck[9] in 1964 reported a 46·7:1 ratio from his clinic population. Ekbom[4] found a 25:1 ratio (Table 2.1).

Table 2.1 Several reports on the incidence of cluster headache and migraine

| Author | Ref. no. | No. patients | | Ratio |
		Migraine	Cluster	Migraine : cluster
Lieder	16	52	4	13·0:1
Carroll	2	89	16	5·6:1
Balla and Walton	1	399	28	14·3:1
Ekbom, K. A.	5	400	16	25·0:1
Lance et al.	15	612	13	47·1:1
Heyck	9	1890	48	39·4:1
Friedman	7	2667	237	11·3:1
Kudrow	—	2835	425	6·7:1

The apparent discrepancies are probably due to several variables. First, there was little standardization of the migraine nomenclature in earlier years, which in some cases were too liberal, and in others, too rigid. Second, migraine may be recognized in several forms; for example, classical, common, hemiplegia, and combination headache. Therefore, depending on the specificity of the migraine diagnosis, ratios could vary significantly. Third, the attraction of more or less migraine or cluster patients to a given clinic would depend on the particular interest of the clinician, house staff, and referring physicians. Last, the incidence of cluster may vary internationally.

Of 4294 patients seen at the California Medical Clinic for Headache from 1971 until 1978, 464 were diagnosed as having cluster, 1000 as having migraine alone, 1835 as having a combination of migraine and scalp muscle contraction headache, and 995 as having other headache diagnoses. Cluster headache patients comprised approximately 10 per cent of the total headache population, yielding a total 'headache' to cluster ratio of 8·3 : 1. The ratio of migraine alone to cluster headache was 2·2 : 1, but when all patients having migraine were included, the ratio became 6·1 : 1 (Table 2.2). Our values were approximately half those of Lieder,[16] Balla and Walton,[1] and Friedman and Mikropoulos.[8] The major reason accounting for our smaller ratio was related to our special interest in cluster headache, attracting a larger patient population with this disorder.

Table 2.2 Relative incidence of cluster headache in a headache clinic population†

Non-cluster headache population			To cluster ($N = 464$)
	N	(per cent)	Ratio
Migraine only	1000	(26)	2·2 : 1
Combination	1835	(48)	4·0 : 1
All migraine	2835	(74)	6·1 : 1
Others	995	(26)	2·1 : 1
Total	3830	(100)	8·3 : 1

† California Medical Clinic for Headache.

We have attempted to estimate the incidence of cluster headache in the general population, having resorted to some liberal extrapolations. Our calculations were based on: (1) the report of Ekbom *et al.*[6] on cluster incidence among 18-year-olds; (2) the age distribution among cluster males in our clinic population (18-year-olds comprised 0·52 per cent of all cluster males); (3) the distribution of 18-year-old males in the general population of the United States (comprising approximately 2 000 000);[3] (4) a constant sex ratio of 5·5 : 1 males to females; and (5) the assumption that all factors concerning cluster headache pertain equally to all geographic areas concerned.

Hence, we have estimated that approximately 400 000 men and 80 000 women in the United States have cluster headache; a prevalence rate of 0·4 per cent for men, 0·08 per cent for women, and 0·24 per cent for both.

These figures probably represent low estimates. Indeed, calculations concerning migraine : cluster' ratios of male populations in headache clinics, in relationship to the prevalence of migraine in the general male population;[19] yields a four-fold estimate for cluster prevalence.

Thus, short of available epidemiological data, we apologetically suggest that from 0·5 million to 2·0 million people in the United States have cluster headache.

Sex distribution

Cluster headache is the only primary headache disorder in which males predominate. Reports of male-to-female ratios vary from 4·5:1 to 6·7:1[4, 8, 13, 17] (Table 2.3). In our series of 425 patients,

Table 2.3   Male:female ratio and mean age at onset of cluster headache

Author	Ref. no.	Patients N	Onset Age	Onset Range	Ratio M:F
Friedman and Mikropoulos	8	50	28	11–44	4·5:1
Lovshin	17	492	—	10–60	6·7:1
Ekbom	4	105	27·5	10–61	5·6:1
Lance and Anthony	13	60	—	8–62	6·5:1
Kudrow	—	425	29·6	1–63	5·1:1

the male-to-female ratio was 5·1:1. When subtyped into episodic and chronic groups, the results were 4·8:1 and 6·3:1, respectively. In this sample, proportionately less women had the chronic variety of cluster headache (Table 2.4).

Table 2.4   Incidence and mean age of onset in cluster headache subtypes

Categories	N	per cent	Mean age of consent
Male			
episodic	280	78·9	29
chronic	75	21·1	33
total	355	100·0	30
Female			
episodic	58	82·9	27
chronic	12	17·1	36
total	70	100·0	28
Both sexes			
episodic	338	79·5	28·6
chronic	87	20·5	33·4
total	425	100·0	29·6

Age of onset

It is generally recognized that the mean age at onset of cluster headache occurs in the late twenties;[10, 12, 14] but may begin at any age.[4, 8, 17] Ekbom[4] reported that the mean age for women was younger than for men. His data has been recently updated to include 208 patients, 180 males and 28 females (Fig. 2.1 from Ekbom, un-

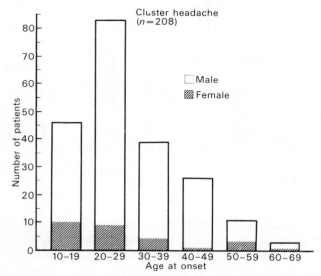

FIG. 2.1 Age at onset distribution of 208 patients with cluster headache. [Unpublished data courteously provided for this publication by Dr K. Ekbom, Dept. of Neurology, Karolinska Hospital and Suder Hospital, Stockholm, Sweden.]

published). Horton[11] reported that in his series, the peak age of onset for episodic patients was in the early thirties, compared to the early forties in the chronic group.

In our series of 425 episodic cluster patients, of whom 355 were males and 70 were females, cluster headache onset, in most cases, began during the third and fourth decades, peaking between 20 to 29 years of age. The incidence rapidly diminished with age, and both males and females shared a similar distribution (Fig. 2.2). Peculiar to the female distribution, an increased frequency occurred between the ages of fifty and sixty years (Figs. 2.1 and 2.2). Confirming Ekbom's[4] and Horton's[11] reports, an older age of onset was found

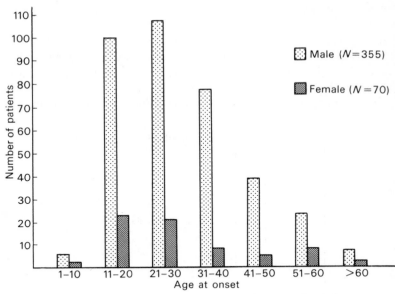

Fig. 2.2   Age at onset distribution of 425 patients with cluster headache.

among chronic patients when compared to those with episodic cluster. Furthermore, the onset of primary chronic cluster headache did not diminish until the sixth decade. In the secondary chronic patients, the distribution pattern is similar to that of episodic cluster, with the exception of increased frequencies in the fifth and sixth decades. The uncharacteristic distribution of the primary chronic group may reflect different aetiologies or pathways. It would also appear that the later the onset of episodic cluster, the greater the chance of it becoming chronic (Fig. 2.3).

The youngest cases of cluster headache have been reported by Lance and Anthony[13] (age 8) and Ekbom[4] (age 8). Since publication of these reports, we have had the opportunity to see in consultation the youngest patient with cluster headache.

Case 1. A three-year, two-month-old girl having a history of headaches since age one, was seen in consultation at the California Medical Clinic for Headache on 14 September 1978. Soon after turning one year of age, the child began to experience left supraorbital-temporal headaches, each morning at approximately the same

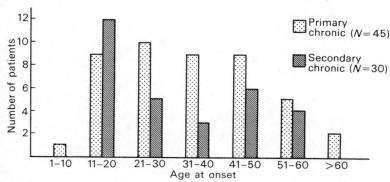

FIG. 2.3 Age at onset distribution of 75 patients with chronic cluster headache.

time. Occasionally, attacks would occur in the middle of sleep and awaken her. Attacks would last approximately 30–40 minutes without medication, and 15–20 minutes, following aspirin. After several months, the headache frequency increased to twice a day, often 12 hours apart. During the attacks, the child was unable to lie down due to increased discomfort, preferring to stand up, or to be held in her mother's arms, pressing the left side of her head against her mother's shoulder. At times, she would lead her mother to carry her outside the house until the attack ended.

Prior to the onset of headache attacks, between ages six and fifteen months, the child exhibited feeding problems and had not gained weight. During this period (age one) the headache attacks began. A neurological examination, EEG, and skull X-rays had been obtained and reported to be within normal limits, prior to our initial consultation. At age three, a second neurological and general examination revealed no abnormalities. The mother was instructed to keep a daily log of headache attacks over a three-week period, paying particular attention to such signs as unilateral lacrimation, rhinorrhoea or stuffiness, and conjunctival injection.

As determined by a daily diary, headaches continued to recur over the left eye. The duration of attacks averaged between 20 and 40 minutes: the shortest, 10 minutes, and the longest, 60 minutes. Over the 21-day period, attacks occurred twice a day for 11 days and once daily for 8 days. She was headache-free for two days during this period (Fig. 2.4). On no occasion did the mother observe rhinorrhoea or conjunctival injection. However, ipsilateral lacrima-

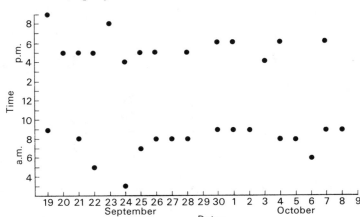

FIG. 2.4   Three-week record of frequency and timing of cluster attacks in a 3-year-old girl (case 1).

tion was noted during some of the attacks. A CAT scan was performed at a later date, the result of which was normal.

The major characteristics of this headache disorder are consistent with the diagnosis of cluster headache; more specifically, primary chronic cluster. The finding of cluster headache in this age group would suggest to all but the most psychoanalytically minded, that psychological factors have little importance in the pathogenesis of this disorder. In the above case presentation, it is likely that the six-month period during which feeding problems and failure to gain weight occurred was related to the development of cluster headache. Had appropriate studies been obtained during that period, perhaps the question of this relationship could have been answered. However, since the cluster attacks appeared rather late in this period, it would suggest that headache was a secondary event.

We are learning that, in cases of anorexia nervosa, hypothalamic dysfunction may be primarily or secondarily related to a 'non-feeding' state, and, as discussed in Chapter 7, hypothalamic dysfunction may be involved in the pathogenesis of cluster headache.

Racial and ethnic distributions

It is not known if cluster occurs in all races and ethnic groups, or if the frequency with which it occurs varies from group to group.

There have been few studies which deal with these questions. Ethnic distributions in clinic populations in the United States, because of cultural and socio-economic factors, do not reflect the actual distribution in the general population.

Realizing these limitations, we surveyed the cluster population at the California Medical Clinic for Headache, for racial and ethnic frequencies, in an attempt to answer the following questions:

1. Is cluster headache found in all major racial and ethnic groups?
2. Quantitatively, are distributions similar for both migraine and cluster populations?
3. Are sex ratios in cluster headache similar for all groups?

The clinic in which the survey was obtained is located in an upper middle class suburban neighbourhood, within the county of Los Angeles, in Southern California. Most of the clinic's patients live within a 100-mile radius of the clinic. In this area, approximately 14 per cent of the general population are non-white,[18] a distribution similar to that for the Jewish population.

Data concerning ethnic origin and race were obtained from 356 males and 70 females diagnosed as having cluster headache, and from 409 male patients having headache other than cluster.

We found that cluster headache occurred in all major races and ethnic groups, the latter representing 59 ancestral countries. The majority of the patients were white (94·8 per cent) and, of these, almost one-fourth were Jewish. Black patients comprised 4 per cent of the clinic population; oriental patients, 0·7 per cent; and American Indians, 0·5 per cent. There were no significant distribution differences between migraine and cluster males. However, the incidence of cluster headache among black males were three times that found in migraine headache. Within each group the difference between males and females were not significant. However, proportionally more Jewish and black women had cluster headache than males of these groups, respectively. The male-to-female sex ratios for black patients were 3·3 : 1 and for Jewish patients, 3·8 : 1. The over-all ratio of all groups combined was 5·1 : 1 (Table 2.5).

Comparing ethnic and racial distributions between the general population of Los Angeles and clinic patients with cluster headache, no difference was found among 'majority' groups. In relation to the population distribution of Los Angeles County, black and oriental

Table 2.5   Comparison of racial and ethnic distributions between migraine and cluster patients at the California Medical Clinic for Headache†

| | Distribution (per cent) | | | |
| | Migraine | Cluster | | |
Race or ethnic group	Males ($N = 409$)	Males (356)	Females (70)	Total (426)
Black	1·2	3·7	5·7	4·0
Oriental	0·7	0·8	0	0·7
American Indian	0·7	0·6	0	0·5
Jewish	23·5	22·2	30·0	23·5
All others	73·9	72·7	64·3	71·3
White	97·4	94·9	94·3	94·8
Non-white	2·6	5·1	5·7	5·2

† In Los Angeles.

patients were under-represented in the cluster population and Jewish patients were over-represented (Table 2.6).

Table 2.6   Racial and ethnic distributions of a clinic† cluster population compared to those of Los Angeles County

| | Population (per cent) | |
Racial or ethnic group	Los Angeles County‡	Clinic (cluster)
Black	10·8 §	4·0
Oriental	2·5 §	0·7
American Indian	0·3 §	0·5
Jewish	14·0 *	23·5
All others	72·4 §	71·3
White	86·4 §	94·8
Non-white	13·6	5·2

† California Medical Clinic for Headache.
‡ Approx. 7 million (ref. 18).
§ Ref. 18.
* Statistics, Jewish Federation Council, 1977.

We may conclude from these findings that:

1. Cluster headache occurs in all major races and ethnic groups as represented by our clinic population.
2. Of the non-white cluster population, black patients predominate, particularly among women.

3. There appears to be little difference in group distributions between migraine and cluster populations. However, disproportionately more black patients are represented in the cluster group.
4. Ethnic and racial distributions of the cluster population do not accurately represent the population distribution of Los Angeles county. The increased frequency of cluster headache among Jewish patients, and the decrease frequency noted in non-white groups, probably reflect differences in cultural, social, and economic status. White 'majority' cluster patients are representative of the population distribution of Los Angeles county.
5. In relation to sex differences in cluster headache, males predominate in all groups. The male-to-female ratio differences between groups may be artefactual as a result of numerous variables that are present. The proportionally higher incidence of Jewish and black women among cluster headache patients may indicate a higher diathesis to cluster headache in these groups.

In 1961, Lovshin[17] reported that cluster headache at the Cleveland Clinic was more common among negroes than caucasians. He stated that of 492 cluster patients, 58 (12 per cent) were black; twice the frequency of the black patient population at the Cleveland Clinic (6 per cent). In addition, he found that, among caucasians, cluster headache males predominated in a ratio of 7·3 : 1, compared to 3·5 : 1 for blacks (in our series the male-to-female ratio among black patients with cluster headache was 3·3 : 1). Lovshin[17] also reported that none of the 492 cluster patients were oriental.

Hence, our results tend to confirm Dr Lovshin's findings that black patients, particularly women, appear to be over-represented within a cluster headache clinic population.

References

1 BALLA, J. I. and WALTON, J. N. Periodic migrainous neuralgia. *Brit. Med. J.*, **1**, 219–21 (1964).
2 CARROLL, J. D. Diagnostic problems in a migraine clinic. In *Background to migraine* (ed. J. N. Cumings), pp. 14–24. Heinemann, London (1971).
3 CHANGES IN POPULATION PROFILE BY AGE. *Statist. Bull.* (*Metropolitan Life*), **54**, 8–9 (Jan. 1973).

4 EKBOM, K. A clinical comparison of cluster headache and migraine. *Acta Neurol. Scand. (Suppl. 41)*, **46**, 1–44 (1970).

5 EKBOM, K. A. Nya behandlingsmetoder vid trigeminusneuralgi, Migrän och Horton's syndrom. *Läkartidn*, **62**, 663–71 (1965).

6 EKBOM, K., AHLBORG, B., and SCHÉLE, R. Prevalence of migraine and cluster headache in Swedish men of 18. *Headache*, **18**, 9–19 (1978).

7 FRIEDMAN, A. P. Atypical facial pain. *Headache*, **9**, 27–30 (1969).

8 —— and MIKROPOULOS, H. E. Cluster headaches. *Neurology*, **8**, 653–63 (1958).

9 HEYCK, H. *Der Kopfschmerz* (4th edn.). George Thieme Verlag, Stuttgart (1975).

10 HORTON, B. T. Histamine cephalgia. *Lancet*, **72**, 92–98 (1952).

11 ——. Histaminic cephalgia linked with respiratory infections. *Headache*, **4**, 228–36 (1964).

12 KUNKLE, E. C., PFEIFFER, J. B. JR., WILHOIT, W. M., and HAMRICK, L. W. JR. Recurrent brief headache in cluster pattern. *Trans. Amer. Neurol. Assoc.*, **77**, 240 (1954).

13 LANCE, J. W. and ANTHONY, M. Migrainous neuralgia or cluster headache? *J. Neurol. Sci.*, **13**, 401–14 (1971).

14 —— and ——. Some clinical aspects of migraine. *Arch. Neurol.*, **15**, 356 (1966).

15 ——, CURRAN, D. A., and ANTHONY, M. Investigations into the mechanism and treatment of chronic headache. *Med. J. Aust.*, **2**, 909–914 (1965).

16 LIEDER, L. E. Histaminic cephalgia and migraine. *Ann. intern. Med.*, **20**, 725–59 (1944).

17 LOVSHIN, L. L. Clinical caprices of histaminic cephalgia. *Headache*, **1**, 3–6 (1961).

18 SERIES PC (1)B₆[1970 CENSUS] GENERAL POPULATION CHARACTERISTICS. US Dept. of Commerce, Washington, DC (1971).

19 WATERS, W. E. and O'CONNOR, P. J. In *Background to migraine* (ed. J. N. Cumings). Heinemann, London (1970).

3 Clinical characteristics

Cluster periods

As noted in Chapter 1, the most frequently encountered form of cluster headache is the episodic type. The 'clustering of attacks' followed by extensive remission periods prompted Kunkle[16] to use the term 'cluster' to describe this entity.

Seasonal frequency

Ekbom[5] reported that 49 of 88 patients (55·7 per cent) experienced their cluster periods mainly in the spring (March–May) and autumn (September–November). In Lance and Anthony's series,[17] of those who considered their bouts as having seasonal predominance, 21 per cent specified spring; 25 per cent, summer; 25 per cent, autumn; and 29 per cent, winter.

At the California Medical Clinic for Headache, the records of 260 cluster patients were surveyed for the month of cluster period onset closest to the initial clinic visit. The greatest number of patients experienced cluster periods in February (13·0 per cent), and June (12·3 per cent). The lowest number was found for the months of November (4·6 per cent) and August (5·4 per cent).

Cluster onsets did not correlate with either the coldest or the warmest temperature. As seen in Fig. 3.1, however, frequency of cluster periods was associated with temperature fluctuations. As temperatures became cooler in winter months (November to February), cluster period frequency increased. In spring, as the climate became warmer, cluster period frequency decreased. As summer heat increased, cluster period frequency increased, but only up to a certain point in early summer. Cooling temperatures in autumn (from September to November) correlated with a decrease in cluster period frequency.

With the exception of a diphasic pattern in summer, cluster period frequency change occurred with seasonal-temperature change. The duration of temperature change, however, was unimportant.

In a second survey, we determined the frequency in which patients would experience time-bound cluster periods, from year to year. Fifty patients were randomly selected from a larger population, whereby

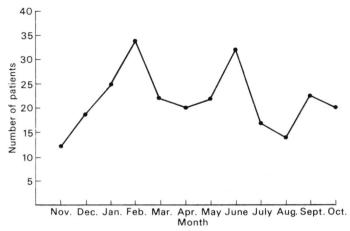

FIG. 3.1   Frequency of cluster period onset among 260 patients plotted against months of the year.

two or more cluster periods had been dated and recorded.

One hundred forty-two cluster periods were recorded for 50 patients. One patient had experienced nine periods, 28 patients each had two periods, and the remainder had from three to six periods, each.

Cluster periods recurred in the same month, in different years, in 8 of 50 patients (16 per cent). In 26 of 50 cases (52 per cent), cluster periods occurred within three consecutive months each year. In the spring months, however, this occurred in only two cases (4 per cent), and in autumn, in four cases. When associated with a given season, cluster periods most often occurred in summertime (24 per cent), particularly in June.

Our data indicates that although many patients will experience cluster periods at a particular time of the year, there appears to be little relationship to spring or autumn.

Frequency and duration

Of 50 patients reported by Friedman and Mikropoulos[8] 54 per cent had at least one attack per year. In a survey of 88 patients, Ekbom[5] found cluster periods occurring less than once a year in 13·6 per cent; once a year, 39·8 per cent; twice yearly, 30·7 per cent; and more than twice a year, 16 per cent.

The duration of these cluster periods varies from 1 to 11 months. (By definition, periods of longer duration are considered chronic.) In our series of 337 episodic cluster patients (of whom 280 were men and 57, women), the median duration of the cluster period was less than two months, confirming the results of others.[5, 8, 16, 17, 20] Approximately 50 per cent of both males and females had cluster periods of a maximum duration of two months, or less (Fig. 3.2).

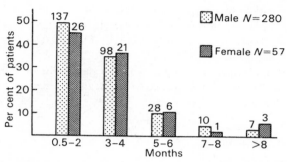

FIG. 3.2   Duration of cluster periods (bouts) in 337 patients with cluster headaches.

In our experience, cluster period durations are surprisingly consistent in a given individual. In some cases, the first cluster period will last less than a week or two, to become more extensive later. Once established, duration of each series is generally maintained. Some individuals, however, may experience an exceptionally long or short period, or the pattern may change completely without apparent reason. We have also found little relationship of age at onset, or duration of disease, to the duration of the cluster periods.

Cluster period precipitation

In some chronic and excessive drinkers there appears to be a paradoxical relationship between alcohol consumption and precipitation of cluster periods. Frequently such patients will report that upon discontinuance of prolonged excessive drinking, a cluster period may begin.

Factors frequently observed in association with the precipitation of cluster periods are reported to be 'stress'[8, 17] and infections or URIs.[11] The causal factors of cluster period induction, however, is no better understood than is the cause of the syndrome. Patients who experience repeated cluster periods for many years remain unable to connect them causally. Experienced clinicians in this area having obtained numerous detailed histories are often frustrated in their attempts to uncover common causal relationships.

In 40 per cent of our patients, the onset of a period has followed such environmental changes as job promotions, workshift changes, moving to a new home, change in routine, travelling, long vacations, or, generally, new situations where the patient must perform well enough to satisfy his peers and himself. We have also found a correlation between cluster period onset to prolonged episodes of rage, anger, 'hurt', frustration, or worry. This relationship is discussed in Chapter 7.

Although our experience suggests that a particular type of stress, as noted above, may be associated with cluster period onset, it remains subjective and speculative.

Remission periods

Duration of remission

A remission is that period where attacks do not occur, either spontaneously or by induction. Remissions have been reported to vary from two months to ten years,[20] having an average duration of less than two years.[5]

Table 3.1   Remission length of 428 male and female patients with episodic cluster headache

Length of remission	Males		Females		Both	
	N	per cent	N	per cent	N	per cent
Months						
1–6	65	18·7	17	21·3	82	19·2
7–12	166	47·7	38	47·5	204	47·7
Years						
2	49	14·1	12	15·0	61	14·3
3	23	6·6	8	10·0	31	7·2
4	18	5·2	1	1·2	19	4·4
5	12	3·4	3	3·8	15	3·5
6–10	9	2·6	1	1·2	10	2·3
11–20	6	1·7	0	—	6	1·4
Total	348	100·0	80	100·0	428	100·0

In our series of 428 patients with episodic cluster headache, remission length was similar for both men and women. The median duration was 7 to 12 months. Sixty-seven per cent of patients had remissions of one year or less, and in 81 per cent, two years or less (Table 3.1). There was no relationship of remission length or cluster period duration to age of cluster onset, or duration of disease.

In our cluster population there were two patients who had experienced cluster periods only twice, 20 years apart. In four others, cluster series occurred at least 11 years apart. Ekbom[5] has followed five patients who were symptom-free, for 11 to 17 years.

The cluster attack

General description

The following is recorded in the first person, and is a vivid and detailed account of a cluster attack. It will provide the reader with an over-all appreciation of the symptomatic, physical, and psychological features of this disorder:

Following a period of perhaps several hours of feeling quite elated and energetic, I experienced a fullness in my ears, somewhat more on the right side than the left, and having a character similar to that which occurs during rapid descent in an airplane or elevator. I then become aware of a dull discomfort, an extension of ear fullness at the base of my skull— further extending over the entire head, on both sides, though somewhat more on the right. At this point, two or three minutes have elapsed; seemingly short but long enough for me to know that a 'cluster' has indeed begun and will ultimately get worse. Such anticipation causes me considerable consternation regarding any decision to continue my activities, or cancel plans and find a place to be alone; giving way to a slowly increasing anxiety, fear, panic, and withdrawal. I become aware of myself 'listening' for changes in my head. Is the cluster prematurely aborting itself, progressing further, or unchanging? A sudden stab, only fleeting, strikes my temple, then again—somewhere near the apex of my skull and upper molars in my face, always on the right side. It strikes me again, deep into the skull base, and as quickly, changes location to a small area above my eyebrow. My nose is stuffed and yet runs simultaneously. If I could sneeze I feel the attack would end. Yet in spite of all tricks, I find myself unable to induce sneezing. While the sharp stabs continue in this fashion, a slow crescendo of dull pain presents itself in an area of a hand's length and breadth over the eye and temporal region. The pain area narrows into a smaller area, and yet, as if magnified, enlarges in intensity. I find myself bending my neck downward, though slightly, as if my head is being gently pushed from behind. My neck, up to the base of my skull, is tight and feels as if I were wearing a neck collar. I feel compelled to remove my tie and loosen my shirt collar even though I know that it will not offer me even a modicum of relief.

In an effort to alter this persistent discomfort, I drop my head between my legs while seated. My face and eyes seem to fill with fluid, but the pain remained unchanged. Despite my suntan, as I look into the mirror, a gaunt, sickly, pale face peers back. My right lid is only slightly drooping and the white of my eye is charted with many red vessels, giving the eye an over-all colour of pink. Right and left pupils appear equal and constricted, as is usual for light-eyed people. Having difficulty standing in one place too long, I leave the mirror to continue alternating my pacing and sitting.

As usual, I am struck with the additional fear that the pain will never end, but dismiss it as impossible since even if that were the case, I would surely kill myself.

The pain, now located somewhere behind my eye and slightly above it, worsens. The pain is best described as a 'force' pushing with such incredible power through my eye that my head appears to be moving backward, yielding to its resistance. The 'force' wanes and waxes, but the duration of successive exacerbations seem to increase. The cluster attack is at its peak which is celebrated by an outpouring of tears from only my right eye. I have now been in cluster for thirty-five minutes—ten minutes at its peak.

My wife peeks into the room where I hold forth. I look up and see her expression of pity, frustration, and helplessness. She sees my tortured face as I have seen it in the mirror at this stage before; a drooling mouth, agape, grey face wet on one side, an almost closed eyelid, and smelling of pain and anguish. She closes the door and leaves, feeling hurt for me, anger for the stupidity of medical science, and guilt—since deep within her mind is the suspicion that she is the cause for my suffering.

I cry for her, but cry more for myself. The pain is so incredible. Suddenly I am overwhelmed by a fury. I lift a chair high over my head and crash it to the floor. With a doubled fist I strike the wall. The pain persists.

Waning periods soon become longer in duration and I allow myself to suspect that the peak is behind me—but cautiously, since I have been too often disappointed.

Indeed, the pain is ending. The descent from the mountain of pain is rapid. The 'force' is gone. Only severe pain remains. My nose and eye continues to run. The road back, as with all travel, covers the same territory, but faster. Stabbing, easily tolerated pain is felt. Then gone. Dull, aching fullness, neck stiffness, all disappear, replaced in turn by a welcome sensation of pins and needles over the right scalp area—similar to the way one's legs feel after it has been 'asleep'. Thus, my head has awakened after a nightmare of torment.

Eye and nose dry, I let out a sigh. I collect my pile of wet tissues that are strewn all over the floor and deposit them in a wastepaper basket. The innocent chair, now uprighted, I rub my slightly bruised fist.

Thus, having ended the battle and cleaned up its field, I open the door and enter my pain-free world—until tomorrow.

Frequency

As reported by various authors, the frequency may range from two attacks per week[5] to eight or more per day.[17] Attacks, however, generally occur with a frequency of 1 to 3 per day.[5] Of Ekbom's series[8] 55·2 per cent of patients, and 50 per cent from Lance's series[17] experienced daily attacks. Approximately 23 to 38 per cent had two attacks, and 13·4 per cent recorded more than two attacks per day[8] (Fig. 3.3).

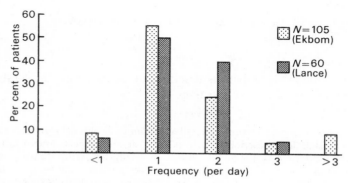

FIG. 3.3   Distribution of attack frequency (per day) in two cluster populations. [From Lance (1978)[17] and Ekbom (1970).[3]]

In our experience, most patients, either at the beginning or ending of their cluster periods, noticed a marked decrease in headache frequency. Cluster periods often 'taper off'. Some had experienced a 'storm' of attacks just prior to the last day of their cluster period. Yet, in others, this 'storm' had appeared suddenly at other times in the period.

Duration

The average duration of headache paroxysms is 30 minutes to 2 hours.[5, 8, 17] This is confirmed by our results from a survey of 500 patients with headaches (428 males and 72 females). Women appeared to have longer attacks than men. Their average duration of attacks was 90 minutes, 30 minutes longer than that of males (Fig. 3.4).

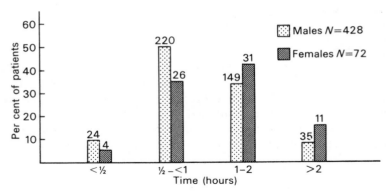

Fig. 3.4   Attack duration among 500 patients with cluster headache.

Pain quality

Most commonly, the pain is described as excruciating, intolerably severe, boring, sharp, or burning.

Lance[17] describes the pain as

> ... particularly distressing. It may be throbbing or pulsating on occasion, but most patients describe the pain as constant and severe. Common adjectives used to describe it are: burning, boring, piercing, tearing and screwing. One patient stated that it was 'like a blunt knife being pushed in, and turned'. Two of our patients said that a dull background pain persisted in the temple or upper jaw between attacks, and four patients mentioned that a dull ache had preceded the bout by some hours, or days. Three patients said that they had sometimes experienced sudden jabs of pain in the affected areas at the time of the headache.

Ekbom and Kugelberg[7] describe the pain quality of the cluster attack as follows:

> the attack started with vague discomfort in the region of one eye, forehead, or temple. Within a few minutes the symptoms became accentuated, assuming the character of real pain. This usually was very intense within ten or fifteen minutes. Thus, at the height of the attack, the pain was constant, excruciating, and generally without fluctuations. Sometimes there were short repeated exacerbations of pain added to the continuous basic headache. This was experienced as severe or very severe, in the majority of patients, and almost intolerable when the attacks reached their peak. Some patients had suffered from other painful conditions, such as ureteric colic, but considered that the headache was equally severe. Typical remarks were that it felt 'as if a knife were being struck into the eye', or 'as if the eye were being forced out', or the like. These severe

attacks usually appeared in the middle of the clusters; the symptoms often being milder at the beginning and the end of the periods.

Friedman and Mikropoulos[8] classified the quality as stabbing, piercing, or knife-like in 56 per cent; throbbing or pounding in 38 per cent, and unqualifiedly sharp in 30 per cent of his patients.

Location

As noted earlier, the attacks are 'always' unilateral; but in some, may change sides from one cluster period (bout) to another. This may even occur during the cluster period, although rarely. In our experience, when cluster attacks change sides, they will be less severe on the side least frequently affected. Ekbom and Kugelberg[7] however, report an exceptional case where attacks occurring on the less involved side became more severe than those on the usual side of attack.

The persistent unilaterality of attacks in 85–90 per cent of all cluster patients contradicts the adage that consistently unilateral head pain is symptomatic of an intracranial mass.

The side predominantly affected in this disorder has consistently been reported as the right (46·8–53·3 per cent).[3, 8, 17] Only 8·3 to 14·4 per cent of patients present with attacks on either side (Table 3.2). With the exception of one case, where attacks occurred bilaterally on a few occasions,[16] there have been no reports of bilateral cluster headache attacks. The site of headache, in order of frequency, has been reported as orbital, 60–89·5 per cent, frontal or temporal, 20–72·4 per cent, and facial including teeth, 12–30 per cent[17, 38] (see Table 3.2 for details).

The following is a case presentation of a patient who, in spite of unmistakable features of cluster headache had a bilateral, occipital pain distribution.

Case 3.1. A 53-year-old man presented with a history of periodic headaches since age 22. Until his most recent period, headaches occurred once a week for a period of two to three months, and were followed by remission periods of one-year duration. His most recent headache period, which differed from previous cycles, began in mid-July and ended in late-August. During this six-week period, he experienced one attack daily, each of one to two hours duration. Attacks always occurred between 4.00 and 5.00 a.m., awakening him from his sleep. The headaches were described as severe, characterized as throbbing and having a bilateral distribution over the occipital

Table 3.2 Location and laterality of pain in cluster headache

Author	Date	N	Location (per cent)					Sides (per cent)		
			Orbital	Frontal	Temporal	Face	Teeth or gingiva	R	L	Either
Friedman and Mikropoulos[8]	1958	50	64	22	28	12		48·6	38·1	13·3
Ekbom[3]	1970	105	89·5	72·4	72·4	12·0	25·7	53·3	38·3	8·3
Lance[17]	1978	60	60·0	46·7	40·0	30·0†	20·0			
Kudrow[15]	1978	423	80·1	68·3	72·3	14·6	18·6	46·8	38·8	14·4

†Cheek area.

and periorbital regions. Nausea and vomiting occurred with each attack, even in the absence of medication. He was unable to lie down during the attack, preferring to pace the floor. He denied other associated symptoms such as lacrimation, rhinorrhoea, nasal stuffiness, or conjunctival injection. He noted that during his susceptible period he was unable to drink alcohol, having recognized it as a provoking agent.

He gave a history of bleeding ulcer disease and 'borderline hypertension'. He uses desiccated thyroid, 6 grains daily. He smokes three packs of cigarettes per day and has recently stopped drinking. His mother suffered with migraine, but neither his father nor two siblings have headache. Physical examination and neurological studies revealed no abnormalities.

Although the diagnosis of this case may be considered cluster-migraine, or atypical cluster, cluster features still predominate. Indeed, this patient responded to prophylactic lithium carbonate, 300 mg, b.i.d., and oxygen inhalation, which effectively aborted most attacks; an effective treatment regimen in cluster, but ineffective in migraine.

The bilaterality and occipital location of pain and the absence of associated symptoms such as lacrimation, rhinorrhoea, and conjunctival injection, are more typical of migraine. His associated nausea and vomiting are not often seen in cluster headache. However, the presentation of daily headache—shortlasting, occurring in a two-month period, and followed by remission—favoured the diagnosis of cluster headache, and more specifically cluster-migraine.

Ekbom and Kugelberg[7] further categorized episodic cluster patients by virtue of pain radiation; either supraorbital (upper syndrome) or infraorbital (lower syndrome). Comparisons between the two groups concerning age onset, laterality and character of pain, affected body positions during attacks, and associated signs and symptoms yielded no substantial differences. The lower syndrome group were somewhat older when clusters first began, and were less likely to experience temporal artery swelling during attacks. Additionally, the lower syndrome group had a significantly higher frequency of peptic ulcer disease (31·0 per cent : 4·3 per cent).

Timing

A major characteristic of cluster headache is the frequency of occurrence of night-time attacks. Quite accurately, Kunkle *et al.*[16]

reported that 20 of 30 patients either always, or commonly, awakened from sleep with the attack in progress. Almost 50 per cent of patients in Friedman's[8] series, experienced their attacks, either more frequently, or only at night. A similar finding of 53 per cent had been reported by Lance.[17]

The most detailed report of cluster headache timing was provided by Ekbom.[5] In agreement with other studies, he found a 62 per cent incidence of nocturnal headaches among 105 patients. Of these, 8.6 per cent were exclusively nocturnal and 53·3 per cent, mainly nocturnal.

Another important feature of cluster headache is the circadian accuracy with which attacks occur. This frequently observed phenomenon is exemplified by the experience of one of our patients. While living on the West Coast his attacks occurred regularly at 7.00 p.m. Following a plane trip east across the United States (time zone difference, three hours later) the timing of his attacks changed to occur regularly at 10.00 p.m. for several days.

In Lance's[17] report, 87 per cent of his patients stated that their attacks were apt to recur at a particular time of the day or the night. Approximately 47 per cent of Ekbom's[5] series experienced attacks with 'clockwise regularity'. This feature, the circadian accuracy of cluster headache attacks, remains unexplained.

A small percentage of patients (7·6 per cent) are reported to experience attacks exclusively during the daytime hours. An additional 34 per cent state, that attacks occur mainly during the day.[8]

Associated features

The cluster headache attack is characterized not only by specific pain quality and pattern, but also associated symptoms and signs, some of which are pathognomonic of this condition. The classical quadrad of associated features are unilateral lacrimation, rhinorrhoea or stuffiness, conjunctival injection, and ptosis. The frequency at which these occur, alone and in combination, is presented in Tables 3.3 and 3.4.

Unilateral lacrimation and injection. Most patients (82–85 per cent) will experience unilateral lacrimation during an attack. It occurs more frequently in association with conjunctival injection, rhinorrhoea or nasal stuffiness, and ptosis; less frequently without either ptosis or injection; and, least frequently, alone (Table 3.4).

Lacrimation is almost always unilateral (bilateral, 5 per cent)[17]

Table 3.3   Frequency of major associated features in cluster headache (50 patients)

Features	Frequency Patients N	per cent
Specific		
Lacrimation	42	84
Conjunctival injection	39	78
Rhinorrhoea (or stuffiness)	36	72
Ptosis	30	60
General		
Photophobia and/or rhinorrhoea	36	72
Occasional or regular nausea (medication?)	27	54

Table 3.4   Frequency of associated feature combinations† in 50 patients with cluster headache

No. of features in combination	Patients N	per cent	Most common symptom combinations	N	per cent
0	2	4·0			
1	1	2·0	Lacrimation		
2	12	24·0	Lacrimation + nasal‡	6	12·0
3	17	34·0	Lacrimation + nasal‡ +conjunctival injection	9	18·0
4	18	36·0	Lacrimation + nasal‡ +conjunctival injection + ptosis	16	32·0

† Excluding nausea and photophobia.
‡ Nasal symptoms include rhinorrhoea and/or stuffiness.

and occurs throughout the attack, with greatest intensity before or during the peak of pain. The affected eye usually becomes engorged with vessels and lends a diffusely red appearance to the eye. Injection may be localized through either the medial or lateral quadrants often sparing the immediate area around the iris.

Unilateral nasal stuffiness or rhinorrhoea. Nasal stuffiness is more apt to occur than rhinorrhoea during the cluster attack. Typically, stuffiness is noted at the earlier stage of, and sometimes prior to, the attack. Some patients who do not experience this symptom may complain that the headache pain is exacerbated by breathing cold air through an unusually patent nostril. Plugging the nostril with cotton is claimed to diminish this pain. When rhinorrhoea occurs, it frequently persists throughout the attack, with or without nasal stuffiness. The nasal discharge is clear and colourless and eosinophile smears are generally negative.

Ptosis. Of 50 patients observed during the cluster attack, 60 per cent developed ipsilateral ptosis. Our observation was similar to that of Ekbom[3] who reported an incidence of 69 per cent; and in addition, miosis was an invariable finding. Lance[17] states that approximately one-third of his patient series exhibited drooping of the eyelid during attacks.

In our experience, ipsilateral lid-lag is a transient feature, occurring specifically with the more intense period of pain. It is completely reversible, occurring only rarely during the interval between attacks. We observed permanent ptosis in only 2 of 400 patients (0·5 per cent) with episodic cluster headache. Ekbom[3] reported an incidence of 5·7 per cent; and permanent ipsilateral miosis in 6·7 per cent of his patients.

Pallor/flushing. The description of a cluster headache as presented by the Ad Hoc Committee on Classification of Headache,[1] includes 'flushing' as an associated sign. Earlier described syndromes such as Möllendorff's[18] red migraine and Bing's[2] erythroprosopalgia, have been confused with cluster headache and has probably contributed to the misconception of flushing in cluster headache. Clearly, Möllendorff described migraine, and Bing, some other related disorder.

Horton *et al.*,[13] in their first publication on 'erythromelalgia', included flushing on the side of the face as a sign. Lance[17] reported that flushing occurred in 20 per cent of his series of 60 cluster patients.

In our experience, flushing has not been a typical feature of the cluster attack. Flushing was not personally observed by Ekbom[3] in any of 45 patients during induced or spontaneous attacks. Actually, ipsilateral pallor appears to be more characteristic of this disorder. In one patient, given nicotinic acid, 200 mg, orally, flushing developed over the *contralateral* side of the face, neck, and upper chest during a severe attack; while the skin region overlying the area of pain was considerably paler than the surrounding skin.[3]

One hundred observations of acute cluster attacks at the California Medical Clinic for Headache did not confirm the presence of a flushing component—except in those cases where patients had applied pressure over the painful area.

Recent results of Doppler flow examination of supraorbital arteries supplemented by facial thermography demonstrated decreased ipsilateral carotid flow during attacks and interim phases in 50 patients with cluster headache.[15]

In a recent editorial in the journal *Headache*, Ekbom and Kudrow[6] stated: 'We had not witnessed a single case where spontaneous flushing accompanied a cluster attack. Numerous patients, however, created redness by persistently rubbing or pressing against the painful facial area.'

Photophobia, phonophobia, and nausea. In our series of 50 patients, photophobia (with or without phonophobia) and nausea accompanied the cluster pain in 72 and 54 per cent, respectively (Table 3.3). Interestingly, the frequency of nausea appeared to be related to the presence of photophobia. Nausea, however, may be a secondary factor; due to pain medication or ergotamine use, or a consequence of anxiety, and not at all related to cluster pain mechanisms.

Other associated signs and symptoms. Lance[17] found a 16·7 per cent frequency of scalp and facial hyperalgesia, occasional or regular vomiting in 28 per cent, and periorbital oedema in 10 per cent of his patients, during the attack. Prominent tender or swollen temporal arteries and veins are reported to occur in 8[3] to 20 per cent[17] of patients.

In our series, three patients complained of focal swelling in an area on the palate. In one case, such a swelling occurred just prior to, or during the attack, itself. In the other two cases, the swelling remained throughout the cluster period. These lesions were observed in two of the above patients on several occasions. (Unfortunately, the quality of photographs obtained were too poor for reproduction.) In both cases, localized swelling was seen on the ipsilateral side of the hard palate in line with the second and third molars. In one case, it was located near the midline of the palate, and in the other, somewhat more lateral. The tissue was soft and blanched easily. The swelling was neither painful nor tender to palpation. This observation supports Lance's[17] finding in 2 of 60 patients, who complained of 'lumps in the mouth' associated with their attacks.

Positions assumed during attacks. We have used as a major criteria of cluster headache the inability of patients to lie still during an attack. When assuming the recumbent position, he will generally writhe with pain, not unlike the behaviour of patients experiencing ureteral colic. This characteristic is peculiar to cluster headache and separates it from other primary headache disorders.

During the attack, the patient is apt to pace slowly or briskly or rock on his feet from side to side, while pressing his hand against the painful area. His head is generally lowered and his posture is slightly stooped during this 'walk'. Not infrequently, especially when awakened during the night, or after several wakeful nights, he may sit in a chair, elbows on his knees, cupping his head in his hands. He may often moan a great deal, cry, or even scream.

As described earlier in this chapter, the cluster patient may strike the floor or wall with his hand or head. (We have two patients who had fractured bones in their hands in this manner.) In some patients prolonged excruciating attacks not infrequently led to moderately severe hysteria associated with hyperventilation and confusion.

Ekbom[3] studied body positions assumed during the headache attack. He reported that of 105 patients, only three (2·9 per cent) were able to lie still. Fifty-eight per cent preferred to walk about, 28 per cent assumed sitting positions, and 10 per cent preferred the recumbent position, although they were unable to remain still.

On rare occasions patients may become violent. In our experience, such behaviour has been limited to younger men. Graham (in a personal communication) tells of a patient who committed homicide during a cluster attack.

Most patients threaten suicide. In our population of 500 patients, only one took an overdose of barbiturates in an attempt to commit suicide. The attempt was made during his remission period. Horton[13] states that his patients had to be watched for fear of suicide, and most were willing to undergo any operation to relieve their pain.

Provocation of attacks

Histamine

Horton *et al.*[13] concluded that vasodilatation was responsible for the symptoms of the cluster headache. Suspecting that this event was histamine-mediated, they tested and successfully induced 'full-blown' attacks in susceptible patients following a subcutaneous injection of histamine, 0·3–0·5 mg. In later publications, he reported success in 69 per cent of his cases with histamine provocation.[10, 12] Subsequently, similar results were reported by one investigator[19] but could not be reproduced by another.[20]

Nitroglycerin

It was not until Ekbom's[4] detailed study, that nitroglycerin became an important experimental tool in this condition. A summary of his findings are as follows:

During the course of their cluster periods, headache was induced in 38 males using nitroglycerin, 1 mg, sublingually, and repeatedly elicited, using the same dosage. Attacks were significantly more severe if testing was done in the middle of the cluster period, rather than near the end. The attack occurred 30 to 50 minutes following administration of the test dose. Nitroglycerin did not provoke attacks if administered a few hours following a preceding attack, or in patients in remission. Administration of an antiserotonin agent prior to nitroglycerin provocation, blocked the attack in only two patients. Anticholinergic administration before induction, blocked the associated symptoms but had little effect on the pain.[4]

Alcohol

In his original observation of 84 patients, at the Mayo Clinic, Horton *et al.*[13] reported that a relationship of alcohol and beverages to exacerbation of attacks was evident. Subsequently, others reported that alcohol had consistently induced cluster attacks.[8, 16, 17, 20]

In a survey of 34 patients and 80 controls, we found the incidence of alcohol consumption significantly greater in the former group ($p < 0.001$).[14] In almost all cases, at the onset of a new cluster period, patients would discontinue alcohol beverages. Although attacks may not be induced with every drinking event, it occurs frequently enough to allow patients to make this association.

It does not require a large or even moderate quantity of alcohol to induce an attack. Many patients report that less than an ounce of whiskey, wine, or beer may provoke attacks. This effect of alcohol is limited to the cluster period and will rarely induce attacks during remission periods.

References

1 AD HOC COMMITTEE ON CLASSIFICATION OF HEADACHE. *J. Amer. med. Assoc.*, **179**, 717–18 (1962).
2 BING, R. Uber traumatische Erythromelalgie und Erythroprosopalgie. *Der Nervenartz*, **3**, 506–12 (1930).

3 EKBOM, K. A clinical comparison of cluster headache and migraine. *Acta Neurol. Scand. (Suppl.)*, **4146**, 1–48 (1970).

4 ——. Nitroglycerin as a provocative agent in cluster headache. *Arch. Neurol.*, **19**, 487–93 (1968).

5 ——. Pattern of cluster headache with a note on the relation to angina pectoris and peptic ulcer. *Acta Neurol. Scand.*, **46**, 225–37 (1970).

6 —— and KUDROW, L. Facial flush in cluster (editorial). *Headache*, **19**, 47 (1979).

7 —— and KUGELBERG, E. Under and lower cluster headache (Horton's syndrome). In *Brain and mind problems*, pp. 482–9. *Pensiero Sci. Publ.*, Rome (1968).

8 FRIEDMAN, A. P. and MIKROPOULOS, H. E. Cluster headache. *Neurology*, **8**, 653–63 (1958).

9 GARDNER, W. J., STOWELL, A., and DUTLINGER, R. Resection of the greater superficial petrosal nerve in the treatment of unilateral headache. *J. Neurosurg.*, **4**, 105–14 (1947).

10 HORTON, B. T. Histaminic cephalgia (Horton's headache or syndrome). *Maryland med. J.*, **10**, 178–203 (1961).

11 ——. Histaminic cephalgia linked with upper respiratory infections. *Headache*, **4**, 228–36 (1964).

12 ——. The use of histamine in the treatment of specific types of headache. *J. Amer. med. Assoc.*, **116**, 377–83 (1941).

13 ——, MCLEAN, A. R., and CRAIG, W. M. A new syndrome of vascular headache: results of treatment with histamine: preliminary report. *Mayo Clin. Proc.*, **14**, 257–60 (1939).

14 KUDROW, L. Physical and personality characteristics in cluster headache. *Headache*, **13**, 197–202 (1974).

15 ——. Thermographic and Doppler flow asymmetry in cluster headache. Presentation 2nd International Migraine Symposium, London (Sept. 1978).

16 KUNKLE, E. C., PFEIFFER, J. B., WILHOIT, W. M., and HAMRICK, L. W. JR. Recurrent brief headache in cluster pattern. *Trans. Amer. Neurol. Assoc.*, **77**, 240–3 (1952).

17 LANCE, J. W. *Mechanism and management of headache* (3rd edn.). Butterworths, London (1978).

18 MÖLLENDORFF. Über Hemikranie. *Virchow's Arch. Path. Anat.*, **41**, 385–395 (1867).

19 PETERS, G. A. Migraine: diagnosis and treatment with emphasis on the migraine-tension headache: provocation tests and use of rectal suppositories. *Mayo Clin. Proc.*, **28**, 673–86 (1953).

20 SYMONDS, C. A particular variety of headache. *Brain*, **79**, 217–32 (1956).

4 Habits, and physical, personality, and occupational characteristics

Physical characteristics

In 1969 and 1972, Graham[7, 8] described certain facial features characteristic of cluster patients. These included ruddy complexion, multi-furrowed and thick 'orange-peel' skin, telangiectasia, narrowed palpebral fissures, asymmetric facial creases, and a broad, prominent chin. These characteristics lend a rugged, masculine look to the cluster individual. Graham[8] characterized this appearance as 'leonine' (Table 4.1). He also reported that patients with cluster headache had unusually broad skulls. This was confirmed by Ekbom and Greitz.[5] who concluded that, independent of sex, most patients with cluster headache had fairly wide skulls.

Table 4.1   Physical characteristics often observed among cluster males

---

Facial
Ruddy complexion
Deep furrows
'Orange peel' skin
Telangiectasia
Narrowed palpebral fissures
Asymmetric creases
Broad chin, skull
Leonine appearance

General
Rugged appearance
Tall, trim
Obesity rare
Hazel eye colour (1/3)

In our clinic, paramedical workers had noted that cluster men were often identifiable by traits other than facial features. Most prominent of these were stature and physique. In order to determine whether cluster males were indeed taller than other male patients in our clinic, we compared heights between the two groups. Other traits were also assessed, including weight, eye colour, haemoglobin level, smoking incidence and frequency, alcohol use, and personality characteristics. A part of this investigation had been published earlier.[11]

Only males were evaluated for height, weight, and haemoglobin values. Height and haemoglobin values were compared with those of male headache controls. Mean weight was established for each of four height ranges, and compared between 240 cluster and non-headache controls. Data on eye colour and smoking and drinking habits were obtained from both sexes. These results were compared to those of headache controls. Black patients were omitted from data collection on eye colour. 'Light' eye colour included grey, green, or blue. Daily alcohol use of at least 3 ounces of whisky, 50 ounces of beer, or 12 ounces of wine was considered moderate to excessive. Significant differences between groups were established by: chi-square (eye colour distribution and incidence of smoking and drinking); t test (height, haemoglobin, and number of cigarettes smoked per day).

Stature and weight

The mean height of 240 cluster males was significantly greater than that of 90 control males (2·5 inches, $p < 0·01$) (Table 4.2); and as earlier reported, significantly taller than the average for American males.[17]

Table 4.2   Mean height of cluster and non-cluster headache males

Group	N	Mean height (in)
Cluster	240	71·0†
Control‡	90	68·5

† $p < 0·01$.
‡ Mixed headaches.

Table 4.3   Mean weight and height compared between 240 cluster males and control group

Mean height range (inches)	N	Mean weight (pounds)	
		cluster	controls†
66–68	41	152	159
69–71	89	166	173
72–74	87	182	185
75–77	23	199	‡

† Metropolitan Life Insurance Co.—ordinary policy holders, 1972–3, (N not given).
‡ Not available.

There was no difference in weight between cluster and control groups, but, in all cases, the mean weight in cluster groups was three to seven pounds less than that of control groups (Table 4.3). Significant differences were not tested since the total number was not provided for control groups; nor was mean weight given for the last height range. Furthermore, in contrast to cluster patients, control subjects were weighed and measured while fully dressed.[16]

Haemoglobin

Haemoglobin values between cluster and control groups were similar; 15·5 mg/100 ml and 15·4 mg/ml, respectively (Table 4.4).

Table 4.4 Mean haemoglobin values of cluster and non-cluster headache male groups

Group	N	Mean Hb (mg/100 ml)
Cluster	100	15·5
Control	50	15·4

Eye colour

A significantly higher frequency for hazel eye colour and lower frequency for light eye colour was found in the cluster group. The frequency of brown eye colour was similar for both groups (Table 4.5).

Table 4.5 Eye colour distribution in cluster and non-cluster headache populations

Group	N	Eye colour (per cent)		
		Light	Hazel	Brown
Cluster	307	41†	23‡	36
Control	300	58	9	33

†$p < 0.01$. ‡$p < 0.001$.

Cigarette smoking and alcohol use

Significantly more patients with cluster headache smoked cigarettes and used alcohol in comparison to control groups ($p < 0.01$ and 0.05 respectively). Number of cigarettes smoked per day and frequency of moderate to excessive drinking was significantly greater among cluster patients ($p < 0.01$ and 0.001, respectively), as seen in Table 4.6.

Table 4.6   Incidence and frequency of cigarette smoking and alcohol use among cluster and non-cluster headache patients

Group	N	Cigarette smoking		Alcohol use (per cent)	
		Smoke (per cent)	No. of cig/day	Drink	Mod–excess
Cluster	280	78‡	33‡	78†	51§
Control	280	52	21	61	19

†$p < 0.05$.   ‡$p < 0.01$.   §$p < 0.001$.

The results confirm those of an earlier study in which cluster men were found to be significantly taller than non-cluster male patients.[11] In another report by Ekbom and Lindahl[4] which concerned calculation of physical work capacity, heights of cluster patients were presented. The mean height of their group was 72 inches. Schéle, Ahlborg, and Ekbom[14] compared this value to that of 55 non-cluster males from the same geographical region; their mean height was $1\frac{1}{2}$ inches shorter.

Increased haemoglobin values were not found in our survey of cluster patients. This confirms the findings of Schéle *et al.*[14] who reported normal haematocrit values among their cluster subjects. These results are in contradiction to our earlier findings, in which we surveyed a small population of cluster patients and found a higher haemoglobin value when compared to controls. Graham, Rogado, Rahman, and Gramer[9] also reported that haematocrit values were elevated in cluster headache patients.

As noted in our earlier report, the frequency of hazel eye colour was significantly higher among cluster patients when compared to controls.[1] This finding is confirmed by our recent survey. It is curious and difficult to interpret. The genetics of eye colour appears to be multifactorial and possibly sex linked. Since the frequency of brown eye colour was similar for both cluster and control groups, the difference in hazel eye colour frequency has greater significance. It may be associated with our finding of a decreased blue eye frequency, and may suggest some defect in melanin regulation in patients with cluster headache.

Cluster headache individuals have been reported to be heavy

smokers. This was confirmed by our earlier[11] and present findings. When compared to controls, a greater percentage of our cluster patients smoked cigarettes, and smoked more, per day. Our findings regarding alcohol use were similar. More cluster patients drank, and drank more, than controls. In comparison of earlier findings, these results indicate that since 1974 there has been a general decrease in the incidence of smoking, not only in cluster headache patients, but in controls as well. Alcohol consumption was also lower than we had previously found. The differences between cluster and control groups, however, remain significant.

Cigarette smoking and alcohol use are habits which appear to be related to personality and psychological factors, and probably play no part in the aetiology of cluster headache. It may be, however, that the observed skin wrinkling, telangiectasia, and other features of the cluster facies, are secondary to excessive cigarette smoking and alcohol use. The relationship between cigarette smoking and skin wrinkling has been reported.[2]

Personality and psychological factors

Graham[8] described cluster males as 'mice living inside of lions'. He suggested that such individuals have difficulty living up to their commitments, and in an effort to do so, experience breaking points, studded with bursts of headache. He pictures the cluster male as a timid individual who has strong hysterical streaks, increased dependency needs, and responds in an exaggerated manner to pain, yet needs to appear manly. He describes this paradoxical picture of a husky male patient who is usually brought to the doctor by his petite but powerful wife, who also makes all appointments, fills all prescriptions, and reports on her husband's condition to the doctor, by telephone.

Our experience with cluster patients differs somewhat, from the above description. It is neither unusual nor infrequently encountered that men, cluster or otherwise, take a subordinate position to their wives in respect to household mechanics and decisions which include doctors' appointments and the filling of prescriptions. It is not unlikely that wives of non-cluster males would have the same opinion of their husbands 'weaknesses' as wives of cluster males. Friedman and Mikropoulos[6] described their cluster patients as ambitious, efficient, and overconscientious, striving for perfection, and having a strong tendency towards compulsive behaviour. They felt that in spite of positions of responsibility, such patients were insecure and generally revealed a lack of self-confidence. Paradoxically, they observe that in spite of loss of sleep, pain, and increased stress, cluster men continue to work.

The personality characteristics of thirteen patients with cluster headache were defined by the Cattell 16 PF test and reported in 1974.[11] Five of sixteen personality factors distinguished the cluster group. These included factors A, G, Q2, Q3, and Q4. A description of these personality characteristics and values for statistical significance is presented in Table 4.7.

Table 4.7   Results of 16 PF testing. Comparison of mean sten scores of 13 cluster headache patients and expected mean sten (5·5)

Factor	Mean sten	Personality characteristics
A	4·3†	Reserved, stiff, detached, critical
B	6·7	
C	5·1	
E	5·9	
F	5·1	
G	7·1§	Conscientious, persistent, staid, moralistic
H	4·7	
I	6·2	
L	5·9	
M	5·7	
N	5·7	
O	5·9	
Q1	6·2	
Q2	7·5‡	Self-sufficient, prefers own decisions, resourceful
Q3	6·9†	Controlled, socially precise, compulsive
Q4	7·1‡	Tense, frustrated, driven overwrought

† $p < 0.05$.   ‡ $p < 0.01$.   § $p < 0.001$.

Concerning the Minnesota Multiphasic Personality Inventory (MMPI) Test, Harrison[10] stated that conversion 'v' patterns were consistently found in all headache patients, including cluster. Steinhilber, Pearson, and Rushton[15] found that cluster patients had scored similarly to an 'other headache' group on all scales of the MMPI. Both groups scored significantly high on the *hypochondriasis* and *hysteria* scales and lower on the *depression* scale. Rogado, Harrison, and Graham[13] obtained similar results in comparing MMPI profiles between 50 cluster patients and matched migraine groups. Both headache groups scored significantly higher than controls on *hysteria, psychasthenia* (obsessive-compulsive), and *hypochondriasis* scales. These groups did not differ from controls when compared for *depression*. In addition, they found that their cluster patients scored above the control group on the scale for *psychogenic lower back pain*.

In 1977,[12] we obtained MMPI results for 41 patients with cluster headaches; 32 men and 9 women. This group was compared to five other headache groups; migraine, combination headache (migraine + scalp muscle contraction headache), post-traumatic cephalgia, conversion cephalgia, and chronic scalp muscle contraction headache. A control group of 30 non-headache subjects was included. With the exception of the conversion group, the mean ages of all other groups were similar (Table 4.8).

Table 4.8 Number of patients, sex, and mean age by diagnostic classification

Diagnosis	*N*	Mean age	Diagnosis	*N*	Mean age	Diagnosis	*N*	Mean age
Migraine			*Combination*			*P-T‡*		
Males	17	38·5	Males	20	38·2	Males	15	41·4
Females	32	36·7	Females	32	35·7	Females	15	39·3
Mean,			Mean,			Mean,		
total	49	37·3	total	52	36·7	total	30	40·4
Cluster			*CSMC†*			*Conversion*		
Males	32	39·8	Males	17	39·1	Males	9	46·1
Females	9	39·4	Females	32	38·0	Females	25	44·2
Mean,			Mean,			Mean,		
total	41	39·7	total	49	38·4	total	34	44·7
Non-headache controls								
Males	15	40·5						
Females	15	40·7						
Mean,								
total	30	40·6						

† CSMC = chronic scalp muscle contraction headache.
‡ P-T = post-traumatic cephalgia.

We found that migraine and cluster groups scored similarly on all scales; and contrary to previous reports, there was no evidence of a conversion 'v' configuration. However, when compared to controls, the male cluster group scored significantly higher on the first three scales (Fig. 4.1). The female cluster group scored significantly higher than controls on only the first (*hypochondriasis*), and sixth (*paranoia*) scales (Fig. 4.2). In disagreement with the results of Rogado, Harrison, and Graham,[13] neither the male nor female

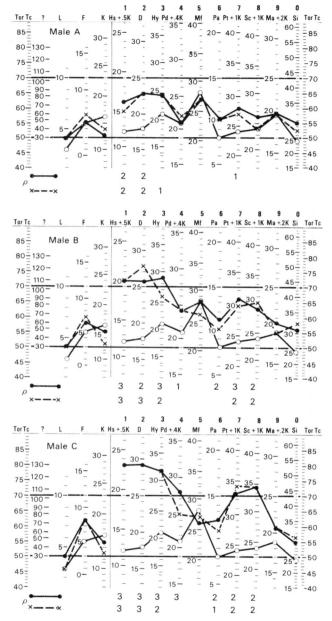

FIG. 4.1   MMPI patterns of male groups A, B, C, and controls, where A = migraine (•———•) plus cluster headache (x - - x); B = combination (•———•) plus chronic scalp muscle contraction headache (x - - x); C = post-traumatic (•———•) plus conversion cephalgia (x - - x); controls (o········o). Included are *p* values of mean score differences between headache groups and controls, where 1 = *p* < 0·05; 2 = *p* < 0·01; 3 = *p* < 0·001. [From Kudrow and Sutkus.[12]]

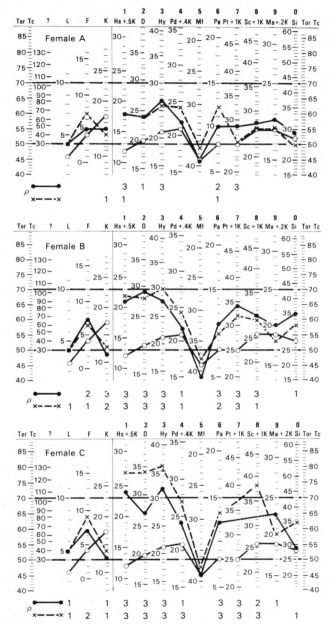

FIG. 4.2 MMPI patterns of female groups A, B, C, and controls, where A = migraine (•———•) plus cluster headache (x - - x); B = combination (•———•) plus chronic scalp muscle contraction headache (x - - x); C = post-traumatic (•———•) plus conversion cephalgia (x - - x); controls (o·······o). Included are *p* values of mean score differences between headache groups and controls, where 1 = *p* < 0·05; 2 = *p* < 0·01; 3 = *p* < 0·001. [From Kudrow and Sutkus.[12]]

groups scored higher than controls on the *PT* (*psychasthenia*) scale

As noted earlier, although cluster patients scored higher than controls on certain scales, no value reached a 'T' score of 65, above which is considered abnormal.

The mean of Five MMPI scales (scales 1, 2, 3, 7, 8) were averaged for a single value of psychopathology. This value was calculated for each headache category including controls, and plotted. As seen in Fig. 4.3, the score for cluster patients did not differ significantly from controls.[12]

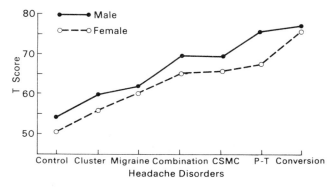

FIG. 4.3   Mean *t*-score values of 5 MMPI scales in each headache disorder. [From Kudrow and Sutkus.[12]]

Occupational status

Cluster headache males are considered to be hard-striving individuals. It is often said that such individuals tend to choose high-powered occupations associated with great responsibility. Yet there have been no studies to confirm these impressions.

We herein report the occupational distribution of 325 cluster males, compared to 200 male controls. The control subjects were husbands of non-cluster headache patients. Excluded from study were students and disabled individuals. Occupations were divided into nine categories, a modification of an occupational classification published in the *Statistical Bulletin*, 1974.[3] Professional, executive, managerial, administrative, and self-employed positions comprised one group. Skilled blue-collar category consisted of such occupations

Table 4.9   Occupational status of cluster males compared to non-headache males

Occupational status	Cluster males†		Non-cluster males‡	
	N	(per cent)	*N*	(per cent)
Professional, executive, managerial administrative, self-employed	121	37·2	72	36·0
Blue-collar (skilled)	73	22·5	36	18·0
Sales	53	16·3	34	17.0
Creative field	25	7·7	10	5·0
White-collar (skilled)	24	7·4	20	10·0
Civil service	11	3·4	11	5·5
Blue-collar (unskilled)	6	1·9	4	2·0
Retired	6	1·9	8	4·0
Unemployed	6	1·9	5	2·5
Total	325	100·2	200	100·0

† Mean age, 39 years.
‡ Mean age, 36 years.

as carpenters, plumbers, machinists, electricians, etc. Heavy equipment operators and other drivers were also included in this category. The creative field category included artists, writers, actors, singers, musicians, and composers. The skilled white-collar category included technicians of all disciplines and other positions requiring special training. The unskilled blue-collar category included labourers and other positions requiring little or no special training. Saleswork, civil service, retired, and unemployed status, were each considered separately. The civil service category included policeman, firemen, and postal workers.

Our results showed that the occupational distribution in both the cluster and control groups were similar. More than one-third of all cluster males and husbands of non-cluster headache women were employed in high-pressure-type, decision-making, responsible positions. This finding and the low employment rate in both groups reflect the socio-economic status of patients attending the California Medical Clinic for Headache. The professional-executive and skilled blue-collar groups accounted for 54 and 60 per cent of all occupations for control and cluster males, respectively.

These data do not support the contention that cluster males tend to select high-pressure, responsibility-loaded occupations. It does not, however, refute the suspicion that job stress, regardless of position, may be greater for cluster men.

The frequency for law enforcement and fire-fighting occupations among cluster males were similar to, and in fact lower than, the control group. This finding does not corroborate the generally held belief that cluster males tend to select dangerous occupations.

Marital status

Curious about the divorce rate among cluster patients, we compared the marital status of 100 cluster males to the same number of male patients having headache conditions other than cluster. Both groups were age-matched; the mean age was 39 years.

Eighty-six per cent of our male cluster patients, between the ages of 21 and 65, were married. This compared to only 64 per cent for the non-cluster group. Of the 86 married cluster patients, 26·7 per cent had been previously divorced. This compares to 17·2 per cent for the non-cluster group.

Table 4.10   Marital status of 100 cluster males and 100 age-matched control males

| | Groups (per cent) | | | |
| | Cluster | | Non-cluster† | |
Marital status	N	(per cent)	N	(per cent)
Married	86	(100·0)	64	(100·0)
Never divorced	63	(73·3)	53	(82·8)
Previously divorced	23	(26·7)	11	(17·2)
Unmarried	14	(100·0)	36	(100·0)
Divorced	6	(42·9)	9	(25·0)
Never married	8	(57·1)	27	(75·0)

† Mixed headache; mean age, 39 years.

Of 14 unmarried cluster males, 57·1 per cent had never been married; the remainder had been divorced. In comparison, the number of unmarried non-cluster males was greater, but not significantly; of these, a greater percentage had no prior marriages (75 per cent).

The most curious finding of this survey is that the marital status of the cluster group was similar to that of the resident male population of the United States; approximately 85·6 per cent of American males between the ages of 25 and 64 are married, and 9·3 per cent are single, having never married.[17] In contrast, the number of unmarried non-cluster males was greater than either of those of the cluster or general populations.

Whether presently married or unmarried, 69 per cent of cluster males, had divorced at least once. This figure was not significantly different for the control group (62 per cent).

It appears from our results that cluster males are not distinguishable from males of the general population, in relation to marital status. Instability, associated with marital and divorce status, is not apparent in our cluster population.

References

1 CARNEY, R. G. Eye color in atopic dermatitis. *Arch. Derm.*, **85**, 17–20 (1962).

2 DANIELL, H. W. A study in the epidemiology of 'crow's feet'. *Ann. Int. Med.*, **75**, 873–80 (1971).

3 EDUCATION AND OCCUPATION AMONG MALES IN THE UNITED STATES. *Stat. Bull. Metro. Life*, **55**, 5–8 (Sept. 1974).

4 EKBOM, K. and LINDAHL, J. Effects of induced rise of blood pressure on pain in cluster headache. *Acta Neurol. Scand.*, **46**, 586–600 (1970).

5 —— and GREITZ, T. Carotid angiography in cluster headache. *Acta Radiologica*, **10**, 177–86 (1970).

6 FRIEDMAN, A. P. and MIKROPOULOS, H. E. Cluster headaches. *Neurology*, **8**, 653–63 (1958).

7 GRAHAM, J. R. Cluster headache. Presentation, International Symposium on Headache, Chicago, Illinois (Oct. 1969).

8 ——. Cluster headache. *Headache*, **11**, 175–85 (1972).

9 ——, ROGADO, A. Z., RAHMAN, M., and GRAMER, I. V. Some physical, physiological and psychological characteristics of patients with cluster headache. In *Background to migraine* (ed. A. L. Cochrane), pp. 38–51. Heinemann, London (1970).

10 HARRISON, R. H. Psychological testing in headache: a review. *Headache*, **13**, 177–85 (1975).

11 KUDROW, L. Physical and personality characteristics in cluster headache. *Headache*, **13**, 197–201 (1974).

12 —— and SUTKUS, B. J. MMPI pattern specificity in primary headache disorders. *Headache*, **19**, 18–24 (1979).

13 ROGADO, A., HARRISON, R. H., and GRAHAM, J. R. Personality profiles in cluster headache, migraine and normal controls. Presented at the 10th International Congress of World Federation of Neurology (Sept. 1973).

14 SCHÉLE, R., AHLBORG, B., and EKBOM, K. Physical characteristics and allergy history in young men with migraine and other headaches. *Headache*, **18**, 80–6 (1978).

52   *Habits, and physical, personality, occupational characteristics*

Where are all the unmarried men?

15 STEINHILBER, R. M., PEARSON, J. S., and RUSHTON, J. G. Some psychological considerations of histaminic cephalgia. *Mayo Clin. Proc.*, **35**, 691–9 (1960).
16 TRENDS AND AVERAGE WEIGHTS AND HEIGHTS AMONG INSURED MEN AND WOMEN. *Stat. Bull. Metro. Life*, **58**, 2–6 (Oct. 1977).
17 Where are all the unmarried men? *Stat Bull Metro Life.* **55**: 9–10, Sept; 1974.

5 Familial and medical histories

Familial history

As reviewed by Ekbom,[10] the incidence of cluster headache among parents of cluster patients is reported to be low. Hence, cluster is not considered to be a genetically transmitted disorder.[28] Studies have shown that among cluster populations of 30 or more patients, the familial cluster incidence ranged between 3·0 and 6·7 per cent. In the same cluster groups, the familial incidence of migraine ranged from 15 to 33 per cent.[3, 8, 9, 10, 33, 38, 43] Lance,[34] in his series of 60 cluster patients, found the familial history of migraine in 22 per cent; none of the relatives had cluster headache. Of 105 cluster patients, Ekbom[10] reported that the familial incidence of migraine and cluster was 15 and 1·9 per cent, respectively.

At our clinic, 495 patients were surveyed for familial incidence of migraine and cluster headache. We obtained two sets of data: the number of cluster patients having parents and siblings with migraine and cluster headache; incidence in the parental population. Positive family histories were recorded separately for each, parent and sibling. Where headache occurred in more than one relative of the same cluster patient, separate groups were formed accordingly in the following combinations: mother plus father; mother plus sibling; and father plus sibling.

Diagnoses of migraine in family members were based on information given by the patients. Parents diagnosed as having cluster headache, were for the most part, personally interviewed or contacted by telephone for confirmation of the diagnoses.

Frequency of positive family histories among cluster patients.

Of 405 males with cluster headache, 27·4 per cent had a positive history of migraine in only one parent or sibling. This compared to 37 per cent of 90 female cluster patients. Of the male cluster group, 10·6 per cent had two or more relatives with migraine headache. This compared to 21·2 per cent for the female cluster group (Table 5.1).

Three per cent of cluster males and 2·2 per cent of cluster females reported a positive family history of cluster in only one relative; 0·6 per cent of the males and 7·8 per cent of the females reported a positive family history of cluster in more than one relative (Table 5.1). The differences between male and female cluster patients were not significantly different. As expected, familial migraine occurred with a frequency considerably greater than that of familial cluster, in both patients' sexes.

Table 5.1 Number of cluster patients having relatives with migraine or cluster headaches

	Cluster patients							
	Males ($N = 405$)				Females ($N = 90$)			
	Migraine		*Cluster*		*Migraine*		*Cluster*	
	N	(per cent)	N	(per cent)	N	(per cent)	N	(per cent)
Occurring in one relative								
Mother	66	16·3	1	0·3	19	21·1	0	0
Father	15	3·7	7	1·7	10	11·1	0	0
Siblings	30	7·4	4	1·0	5	5·6	2	2·2
Subtotal	111	27·4	12	3·0	34	37·8	2	2·2
Occurring in > 1 relative								
Mother + father	11	2·7	0	0	5	5·6	1	1·1
Mother + siblings	24	5·9	1	0·3	14	15·6	1	1·1
Father + siblings	8	2·0	1	0·3	0	0	5	5·6
Subtotal	43	10·6	2	0·6	19	21·2	7	7·8
Total	154	38·0	14	3·5	53	58·9	9	10·0

Parental migraine was found in 30·6 per cent of 405 male cluster patients. This was not significantly different from 53·3 per cent of female cluster patients. In all, 172 (34·8 per cent) of 495 patients gave a parental history of migraine. The figures were considerably lower for a parental history of cluster headache in both patients' sexes. Among male patients only 2·5 per cent had parents with cluster headache and cluster headache was found in fathers more times more often than in mothers. Among women patients 7·8 per cent had parents with cluster headache, and as with male patients, fathers were most often involved. Considering patients' sexes together, 34·8 per cent gave a parental history of migraine, and 3·4 per cent, cluster headache (Table 5.2).

Incidence of migraine and cluster headache in the parental population

The incidence of migraine among 810 parents of cluster headache

Table 5.2 Number of cluster patients having parents with migraine or cluster headaches

	Cluster patients											
	Males (N = 405)				Females (N = 90)				Total (N = 495)			
	Migraine		Cluster		Migraine		Cluster		Migraine		Cluster	
Parent	N	(per cent)	N	(per cent)	N	(per cent)	N	(per cent)	N	(per cent)	N	(per cent)
Mother	90	22·2	2	0·5	33	36·7	1	1·1	123	24·9	3	0·6
Father	23	5·7	8	2·0	10	11·1	5	5·7	33	6·7	13	2·6
Both	11	2·7	0	0	5	5·6	1	1·1	16	3·2	1	0·2
Total	124	30·6	10	2·5	48	53·3	7	7·8	172	34·8	17	3·4

males was 135 (16·7 per cent). The majority was found among mothers (24·9 per cent). Only 10 out of 810 parents were recorded as having cluster headache (1·2 per cent). This disorder occurred with a fourfold frequency in fathers (2·0 per cent). As expected, the lowest incidence of cluster headache among parents, were found in mothers (0·5 per cent); the lowest incidence of migraine occurred in fathers (8·4 per cent) (Table ⸗

Table 5.3   Incidence of migraine and cluster in parents of 405 male cluster patients

Parents	N	Migraine		Cluster	
		N	(per cent)	N	(per cent)
Mothers	405	101	24·9	2	0·5
Fathers	405	34	8·4	8	2·0
Total	810	135	16·7	10	1·2

Of 180 parents of women cluster patients, 29·4 per cent had migraine headache and 4·4 per cent had cluster headache. As with the parents of male patients, migraine was more prevalent among mothers, whereas cluster headache occurred more frequently among fathers (Table 5.4).Of 990 parents of all cluster patients combined,

Table 5.4   Incidence of migraine and cluster in parents of 90 women cluster patients

Parents	N	Migraine		Cluster	
		N	(per cent)	N	(per cent)
Mothers	90	38	42·2	2	2·2
Fathers	90	15	16·7	6	6·7
Total	180	53	29·4	8	4·4

188 (19 per cent had migraine headaches; 28·1 per cent were found among mothers and 9·9 per cent among fathers. Eighteen parents (1·8 per cent) had cluster headaches; 0·8 per cent were mothers and 2·8 per cent were fathers (Table 5.5).

Including siblings, a positive family history of migraine was found in 41·8 per cent of our total cluster population. This figure is considerably higher than the figure reported by Lance (21·7 per cent),[34] Ekbom (15·2 per cent),[10] and others, [2,8,9,22,38] but similar to those

Table 5.5   Incidence of migraine and cluster in parents of 495 cluster patients (male and female)

Parents	N	Migraine		Cluster	
		N	(per cent)	N	(per cent)
Mothers	495	139	28·1	4	0·8
Fathers	495	49	9·9	14	2·8
Total	990	188	19·0	18	1·8

of Bickerstaff,[3] Dalsgaard-Nielsen (52 per cent),[6] Kunkle (33 per cent),[33] and Symonds (35 per cent).[45]

Of 105 cluster patients, Ekbom[10] found two relatives with cluster headache (1·9 per cent); Lance[34] found none, in his series of 60 cluster patients. In our series, 4·7 per cent of our patients, gave a positive family history of cluster headache. This result is in agreement with others.[2,3,8,33,38]

Concerning the incidence of migraine among parents of cluster headache patients, Ekbom[10] reported that of 210 parents, 4·8 per cent were migraineurs. This is lower than our result of 19 per cent. Graham[23] found that 17 per cent of relatives of cluster patients, including siblings, had migraine. He also reported that of 377 relatives, including siblings, 6 per cent had cluster headache;[23] higher than our result of 1·8 per cent.

Regarding sex differences, among parents and siblings with cluster headache, males appear to predominate.[3,8,10,43] In our present series, cluster headache occurred in fathers in a ratio of 3–4:1, regardless of the patients' sex. Among parents with migraine, mothers predominated by a ratio greater than 2·5:1.

Conclusions

Considering all available evidence, a positive family history of migraine among cluster patients varies between 15 and 20 per cent; 19 per cent in the present series. The incidence of familial migraine among cluster patients differs little from the familial incidence in control populations. The latter varies between 11 and 17 per cent;[10,19,36,44] hence, it would appear that migraine genetics plays little role in cluster headache. It is also unlikely that cluster headache is genetically transmitted, since the incidence of this disorder among parents of cluster patients is small, 2 to 6 per cent.

Finally, it should be noted that widely disparate data concerning the familial incidence of migraine and cluster, in cluster headache populations, are probably due to: varied numbers and sex distributions of surveyed populations; inadequate patient reporting; and, inconsistent criteria for the diagnosis of migraine in relatives.

HLA antigens in cluster headache

HLA antigens, occurring with increased frequency in specific disorders, are considered genetic markers. In this regard, classical migraine and cluster headache was of particular interest. We selected 25 male cluster and 18 female migraine patients in search of HLA antigens specificity.

Typing for 26 HLA antigens in the cluster group and 29 HLA antigens in the migraine group was performed by the Microdroplet Lymphocytic Cytotoxicity Test, in the laboratory of Dr Paul I. Terasaki at UCLA. The chi-square test was used to determine statistical significance. The p value was corrected by multiplying it by the number of comparisons. As such, chi-square of 8·0 or greater would indicate significant difference.

HLA 13 appeared to be associated with classical migraine before correction ($p < 0.05$). However, after the correction (p value times number of specificities), significance was not obtained. Therefore, no significant differences in HLA antigen frequency were found in either the cluster or migraine groups when compared to controls (Tables 5.6 and 5.7). We concluded that if genetic factors are associated with cluster headache or classical migraine syndromes, such an association is outside the HLA histocompatibility antigen system.

Past or current medical history

Coronary artery disease

In 1968, Graham[25] described a patient who experienced relief of intermittent claudication, only during spontaneous cluster attacks.

Ekbom[14] in 1970, observed that in one patient, a distinct reduction of anginal attacks occurred during several cluster periods. This patient was subjected to several physiological tests; and the results were reported in 1971.[18] He had experienced angina and episodic

Table 5.6 Frequency of HL-A antigens in cluster headache males

Antigens	Controls (N = 1085) (per cent)	Patients (N = 25) (per cent)	χ^2	Antigens	Controls (N = 1085) (per cent)	Patients (N = 25) (per cent)	χ^2
HL-A1	28	32	0·0002	HL-A8	20	16	0·0004
HL-A2	48	52	0·0002	HL-A12	27	16	0·4030
HL-A3	27	40	0·5061	HL-A13	5	4	0·2370
W23	3	8	0·3058	TE 50	17	16	0·0742
W 24	24	16	0·1453	W 22	4	8	0·0010
HL-A10	13	12	0·0935	W 27	8	12	0·0006
HL-A11	12	0	1·5008	W 14	8	12	0·0006
W 28	7	4	0·0154	W 15	11	4	0·1920
W 29	7	8	0·1482	W 17	9	8	0·1313
W 30	10	4	0·0972	W 18	8	12	0·0006
W 32	7	4	0·0154	TE 60	13	16	0·0066
HL-A5	10	0	1·0192	W 16	8	12	0·0006
HL-A7	25	20	0·0111	W 21	4	12	0·3271

Table 5.7 Frequency of HL-A antigens in classical migraine

Antigens	Controls (N = 3896) (per cent)	Patients (N = 18) (per cent)	χ^2	Antigens	Controls (N = 3896) (per cent)	Patients (N = 18) (per cent)	χ^2
HL-A1	31	22	0·32	HL-A7	25	11	1·20
HL-A2	47	39	0·20	HL-A8	21	33	0·91
HL-A3	27	33	0·09	HL-A12	26	22	0·01
AW 23	3	6	0·00	HL-A13	4	17	4·79
AW 24	12	22	0·88	HL-A14	9	6	0·00
HL-A10	13	11	0·01	HL-A15	10	6	0·03
HL-A11	12	17	0·08	BW 16	8	17	0·93
HL-A28	8	11	0·00	BW 17	9	0	0·84
HL-A29	7	17	1·42	HL-A18	8	0	0·66
AW 30	10	6	0·03	BW 21	5	0	0·18
AW 31	1	0	0·58	BW 22	4	11	0·82
AW 32	7	0	0·49	HL-A27	7	0	0·49
AW 33	1	6	0·86	BW 35	19	6	1·21
HL-A5	10	11	0·06	BW 37	1	6	0·89
				BW 40	12	17	0·08

cluster intermittently, for periods of 5 and 12 years, respectively. During headache periods he required less nitroglycerin and during remission periods, used this medication up to four times a day. The frequency of anginal attacks in cluster and remission periods occurred in a ratio of 1 : 7–8. Neither seasonal change, psychological factors, physical activity, nor changes in smoking habits explained this difference in anginal frequency. Stress (cycle ergometry) tests and resultant blood-pressure and pulse changes were obtained during cluster and remission periods. The results of these tests were consistent with the observed differences in anginal frequency between periods. That is, during cluster periods, the threshold for provocation of angina pectoris was manifestly elevated during the cluster period, compared to four remission periods. Urine catecholamine levels and monitored cardiac rates obtained during both periods revealed no significant differences.[18]

Ekbom and Lindahl[18] concluded that these observations support the hypothesis of a change in vegetative tone between cluster and remission periods, which affects reactivity of cranial vessels[16] and cardiac function.

Paradoxically, Graham[23] reported that he and Lovshin had noted a higher incidence of coronary artery disease among cluster patients. In this regard, Graham[23] found abnormal lipoprotein patterns in 16 of 23 cluster males. The finding of hyperlipidaemia in cluster headache is quite significant since essential hyperlipidaemia, as described by Fredrickson,[21] is familial and rare. Thus, hyperlipidaemia may be a genetic marker for cluster headache. In support of this view, Oleson[39] described Type 2A and Type 4, essential hyperlipidaemia in two brothers with chronic cluster headache. By history, he determined that the mother also had these disorders. He further screened 11 other cases of cluster headache (5 episodic, 6 chronic) for plasma lipid profiles. Of the 6 chronic patients, 2 had Type 4 essential hyperlipidaemia; and although plasma lipid values among the episodic group were normal, one patient had bilateral xanthelasmata. Although he suggested that lipid deposition on arteries may have aetiological significance in cluster, successful treatment for hyperlipidaemia in one patient did not affect the cluster headaches.

Graham[23] believes that a factor common to angina and cluster is maleness; and reported that of 85 patients with vascular headache who had developed drug-induced fibrosis, 20 per cent had cluster headache. Of 18 patients who specifically developed pulmonary fibrosis, 33 per cent were cluster patients and all were males.

Regarding the incidence of coronary disease in cluster males, we compared the histories of 119 males with cluster to 140 non-cluster headache males. A second control consisted of national prevalence data provided by the American Heart Association.† The mean ages of our male cluster population and controls were 43 and 41 years, respectively.[31]

The incidence of coronary heart disease (CHD) for the cluster group was 7·6 per cent; non-cluster controls, 3·6 per cent; and US male population, 3·0 per cent. The incidence of CHD in the cluster group was twice that of controls but the difference was not significant.[31] Therefore, this survey did not support the contention that cluster males were prone to coronary artery disease. Perhaps, as suggested by Graham,[24] had our groups been older, a significant difference in CHD incidence would have been noted.

Bradycardia associated with cluster headache, was first described by Rosenthal in 1979.[41] Since then this relationship has been described and reported by others.[4, 5, 11, 13, 20, 29, 32, 41]

Jacobson[29] had observed 10 cluster headache attacks in a 64-year-old man, following an acute myocardial infarction. Pre- and post-headache attack pulse rates varied between 52–68/min. During attacks, however, the pulse rate dropped to 40–48/min, while blood-pressure remained constant, or rose by no more than 10 mm Hg. Intravenous atropine, 0·4 mg, affected neither heart rate nor headache. Neither i.v. diphenhydramine 10–15 mg, nor 0·5 ml of saline affected character, quality or duration of pain, or heart rate. During one cluster attack manual compression of the right carotid artery caused a drop in pulse rate to 30–50/min, multifocal paroxysmal atrial contractions, and sinus arrest with supraventricular escape; pain, however, was unaffected. Jacobson[29] concluded that bradycardia during the cluster attack, may be due to integrated parasympathetic discharge involving the brain stem and cranial nerves. It may also result from an oculocardiac reflex due to orbital traction or pressure.

Ekbom[11] reported on ECG and blood-pressure changes in 17 male patients during nitroglycerin-induced cluster headaches. He reported the following:

---

† Estimated prevalence of the major cardiovascular diseases in the US. *Heart Facts 1972*, American Heart Association (1975).

1. Typical cluster headaches resulted 30–50 minutes following nitroglycerin (1 mg sublingually).
2. The mean heart rate was significantly reduced during attacks, as compared to pre-test values.
3. Systolic and diastolic blood-pressures increased significantly during paroxysms.
4. The observed changes in heart-rate and blood-pressure values were proportional to the severity of head pain, most pronounced at the height of attacks and normal at the termination of pain (Fig. 5.1).

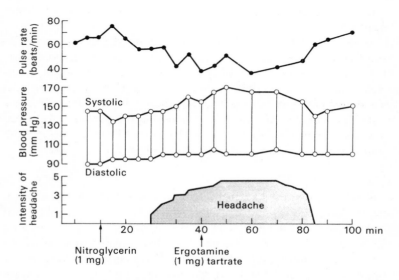

FIG. 5.1 Results of a provocation test with nitroglycerin. Severe attack developed after a latency period of twenty minutes. Note the marked bradycardia and blood-pressure elevation at the height of pain. [Reproduced by courtesy of author, K. Ekbom[11].]

Electrocardiograms in 8 of 17 patients showed P wave changes indicative of increased vagal tone (Fig. 5.2).

From these results, and observations of others, Ekbom[11] postulated that bradycardia during the cluster attack may, in part, be due to an oculocardiac reflex; a reflex mediated through the trigeminovagal pathways.[30,40] He further concluded that the observed increased blood-pressure was probably a response to pain; hence, vagal and

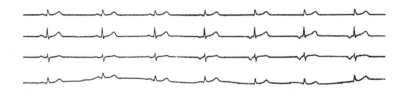

FIG. 5.2   The electrocardiogram during a severe induced attack of cluster headache. Leads, from the top: I, II, III, CR. Note P-wave changes in leads II and III, suggestive of a coronary sinus rhythm. [Reproduced by courtesy of author, K. Ekbom[11].]

sympathetic fibres are activated during provoked attacks of cluster headache.

Bruyn, Bootsma, and Klawans[4] interpreted the occurrence of bradycardia and other phenomena during cluster attacks as evidence for a primary abnormality of autonomic centres in the lower brainstem. They concluded that the concept of 'parasympathetic crisis' as a pathogenetic mechanism in cluster headache is untenable, since it inadequately explains the mixed pressor and depressor effects seen in this disorder. They hypothesized that cluster headache arises from central excitatory and inhibitory alpha adrenergic paroxysms.

Peptic ulcer disease

Several investigators had suspected a possible relationship between peptic ulcer disease and cluster headache.[27, 1, 37] K. A. Ekbom,[15] in 1947, reported a 13 per cent incidence of ulcer symptoms among 23 patients with cluster headache, but had not reported the mean age of this population. Ekbom and Kugelberg,[17] distinguishing upper and lower cluster syndromes, reported an ulcer disease incidence of 2·4 and 25 per cent, respectively; 13 per cent of their total group of 77 patients had a history of ulcer disease. Neither mean age nor sex distribution was given. Subsequently, Ekbom[14] surveyed 89 males with cluster headache and found an ulcer history in 17 per cent; 31 per cent among lower syndrome and 4·3 per cent in upper syndrome patients. Neither the mean age of males, nor control group data were included; however, the mean age of the total group was 39·5 years.

Graham[26] in 1969 and again in 1972[23] reported an ulcer incidence of 20 and 22 per cent, respectively. The control group of 100 migraine patients had a significantly lower incidence of ulcer disease. In both groups, sexes were combined. He also found very high secretion rates of gastric acid, approaching that of Zollinger–Ellison range. Gastric acid secretion was noted to increase markedly during the attack phase and decrease with the cessation of headache.

In 1976[31] we reported the results of a survey for peptic ulcer disease among 119 male and 21 female cluster headache patients. The mean age was 43 years and 46 years, respectively. Age-matched control groups of 140 male and 140 female migraine patients were compared.

Of 119 cluster males, 25 (21·1 per cent) had an early or current history of peptic ulcer disease that was predominantly duodenal. This compared to 10·7 per cent of 140 male migraine controls. The frequency of ulcer disease history in cluster women was significantly different from migraine controls; although both were twice the value estimated for women in general population (2·5 per cent).[31]

More recently, we surveyed 355 male cluster patients and found results similar to our earlier report. The incidence of peptic ulcer disease was 19·7 per cent (Table 5.8).

Migraine

The frequency with which migraine occurs in patients with cluster headache is of special interest, since an aetiological link between the two disorders have been suspected by some, and questioned by others. A finding of a lesser or greater incidence of migraine, however, is equally insignificant to this issue. A lower migraine incidence may suggest 'substitution' and infers that cluster is a variant of migraine. But it may also be interpreted as evidence against a relationship between the two disorders. A high incidence of migraine may argue for a common susceptibility, or pathogenesis.

Ekbom[10] reported that 3 of 105 cluster patients (2·9 per cent) had migraine. In his extended series of 163 patients, he found five (3·1 per cent) with migraine.[12] Lance and Anthony[35] in their cluster series, found that 4 of 60 (6·7 per cent) had migraine headache. Graham[23] reported a 27 per cent migraine occurrence among 84 patients with cluster; and 5 per cent for a non-headache control group of 114 subjects.

In our survey of 140 cluster patients (119 males and 21 females), we found a migraine incidence of 10·9 and 52·4 per cent, respectively.[31] Of the total cluster group, 24 patients (17·1 per cent), had migraine. In comparison to the general population,[7,47] the incidence in cluster males was similar, but in cluster women, considerably

Table 5.8 Frequency of ulcer disease in cluster headache

Author	Sex	Cluster groups				Migraine controls		
		Total N		Ulcer N	History (per cent)	Total N	Ulcer N	History (per cent)
Ekbom, K. A. (15)	Both	23		3	13·0			
Ekbom, K. &								
Kugelberg, E. (17)	Both	36	(lower)	9	25·0			
		41	(upper)	1	2·4			
		77	(total)	10	13·0			
Graham, J. R. (26)	Both	100		20	20·0	100	7	7·0
(23)	Both	100		22	22·0			
Ekbom, K. (14)	Males	42	(lower)	13	31·0			
		47	(upper)	2	4·3			
		89	(total)	15	16·9			
Kudrow, L. (31)	Male	119		25	21·1	140	15	10·7
	Female	21		1	4·8	140	8	5·7
Present series	Male	355		70	19·7			

higher. Our results argue against a relationship between these disorders, since in cluster males (the predominant sex), migraine occurs with the expected frequency for males in general.

Other disorders

The frequency of other disorders occurring in cluster headache has also been reported. Allergy in cluster patients has been reported to occur with a frequency of 12 per cent,[22] 15 per cent,[35] and 22 per cent.[42] These values are probably not significant when compared to control populations.[42] Lance[34] and Symonds[45] reported an incidence of 8·3 and 17·7 per cent of hay fever in cluster patients, respectively. Asthma has been reported to occur in 5 per cent[35] and 11 per cent[42] of cluster populations. A history of head injury has been consistently reported at 11·8 to 16 per cent.[22,35,45]

In an earlier study we reported the frequency of hypertension in cluster headache.[31] Of 119 males, four (3·4 per cent) had hypertension. None of 21 women had this disorder. The incidence of high blood-pressure in the total cluster group was lower, although not significantly lower than control values (8·6 per cent).

Recently, we evaluated 230 male cluster patients with regard to previous medical disorders and surgical histories. Coronary artery disease, ulcer history, and migraine, were excluded. In our group of 230 males, 13·9 per cent gave a history of allergy; in agreement with other reports.[22,35,42] Hypertension was present in only 6·5 per cent, not significantly different from our earlier study (3·4 per cent).[31] A history of significant head injury was given by 5·2 per cent of patients; lower than other reported frequencies.[22,35,45] The incidence of asthma in our cluster group (3·5 per cent) was similar to Lance's and Anthony's results (5·0 per cent).[35]

Regarding surgical procedures, more than one-third of our cluster males had tonsillectomies performed in childhood. 16·5 per cent had surgery for acute appendicitis. Herniorrhaphy was performed in 7·4 per cent; nasal surgery, 4·8 per cent; and disc surgery (cervical or lumbar) in 3·9 per cent of our cluster group.

Most curious was our finding of a high incidence of cancer. Of 230 males, 8 (3·5 per cent) had a current or past history of cancer. This compares to 0·3 per cent of the general male population.[46]

The mean age of our patients was 57·6 years. In two patients, cancer had preceded the cluster onset by many years. One had carcinoma of the colon and the other, malignant melanoma. Six

Table 5.9   Current or previous history of medical and surgical disorders in 230 male
cluster patients

History of other disorders

Medical	N	(per cent)	Surgical	N	(per cent)
Allergy	32	13·9	Tonsillectomy	87	37·8
Hypertension	15	6·5	Appendectomy	38	16·5
Head injury	12	5·2	Herniorrhaphy	17	7·4
Asthma	8	3·5	Nasal	11	4·8
Carcinoma	8	3·5	Disc	9	3·9

patients developed cancer since cluster onset. Of these, one died following surgery for glioblastoma multiformis. All others are alive and well following surgery for prostrate cancer (2), adenocarcinoma of the colon (1), and pulmonary cancer (2).

Of 68 cluster women, one died from an astrocytoma, grade 3, and another, was successfully treated for a benign brain tumour.

The increased incidence of cancer in our cluster population may not be representative of all cluster populations. Our results may have been artefactual. Such a survey should be undertaken by other investigators.

References

1 ALFORD, R. I. and WHITEHOUSE, F. R. Histaminic cephalgia with duodenal ulcer. *Amer. Allerg.*, **3**, 200–3 (1945).
2 BALLA, J. I. and WALTON, J. N. Periodic migrainous neuralgia. *Brit. med. J.*, **1**, 219–21 (1964).
3 BICKERSTAFF, E. R. The periodic migrainous neuralgia of Wilfred Harris. *Lancet*, **1**, 1069–71 (1959).
4 BRUYN, G. W., BOOTSMA, B. K., and KLAWANS, H. L. Cluster headache and bradycardia. *Headache*, **16**, 11–15 (1976).
5 DANDY, W. E. (1931). Treatment of hemicrania (migraine) by removal of the inferior cervical and first thoracic sympathetic ganglia. *Bull. Johns Hopkins Hospital*, **48**, 357–61 (1931).
6 DALSGAARD-NIELSEN, T. Migraine and heredity. *Acta Neurol. Scand.*, **41**, 287–300 (1965).
7 ——. Some aspects of the epidemiology of migraine in Denmark. In *Kliniske aspekteri migraeneforskningen*, p. 18. Nordlundes Bogtrykkski, Copenhagen (1970).
8 DUVOISIN, R. C., PARKER, G. W., and KENOYER, W. L. The cluster headache. *Arch. intern. Med.*, **108**, 111–16 (1961).

9 EADIC, M. J. and SUTHERLAND, J. M. Migrainous neuralgia. *Med. J. Aust.*, **53**, 1053–6 (1966).
10 EKBOM, K. A clinical comparison of cluster headache and migraine. *Acta Neurol. Scand.* (*Suppl.*), **4146**, 1–48 (1970).
11 ——. Heart rate, blood pressure and electrocardiographic changes during provoked attacks of cluster headache. *Acta Neurol. Scand.*, **46**, 215–24 (1970).
12 ——. Migraine in patients with cluster headache. *Headache*, **14**, 69–72 (1974).
13 ——. Nitroglycerin as a provocative agent in cluster headache. *Arch. Neurol.*, **19**, 487–93 (1968).
14 ——. Patterns of cluster headache with a note on the relations to angina pectoris and peptic ulcer. *Acta Neurol. Scand.*, **46**, 225–37 (1970).
15 EKBOM, K. A. Ergotamine tartrate orally in Horton's 'histaminic cephalgia' (also called Harris's 'ciliary neuralgia'). *Acta Psychiat. Scand.* (*Suppl.*), **46**, 106–13 (1947).
16 EKBOM, K. and GREITZ, T. Carotid angiography in cluster headache. *Acta Radiologica*, **10**, 177–86 (1970).
17 —— and KUGELBERG, E. Upper and lower cluster headache (Horton's syndrome). In *Brain and mind problems*, pp. 482–9. Il Pensiero Scientifico Publishers Ltd., Rome (1968).
18 —— and LINDAHL, J. Remission of angina pectoris during periods of cluster headache. *Headache*, **11**, 57–62 (1971).
19 ELY, F. A. The migraine-epilepsy syndrome. *Arch. Neurol. Psychiat.*, **24**, 943–9 (1930).
20 FISHER, J. H. Migraine. *Proc. roy. Soc. Med.* (*Part 3*). *Ophthal.*, **12**, 49–55 (1919).
21 FREDRICKSON, D. S. Disorders of liquid metabolism and xanthomatosis. In *Harrison's Principles of Internal Medicine* (7th edn.), pp. 634–43. McGraw-Hill, New York (1974).
22 FRIEDMAN, A. P. and MIKROPOULOS, H. E. Cluster headaches. *Neurology*, **8**, 653–63 (1958).
23 GRAHAM, J. R. Cluster headache. *Headache*, **11**, 175–85 (1972).
24 ——. Discussion, Bergen Migraine Symposium (June 1975).
25 ——. Proc. conference on cluster headache, *Headache Research Foundation*, Faulkner Hospital, Massachusetts (1968).
26 ——. The physical and physiological characteristics of patients with cluster headache. 3rd International Symposium on Migraine, London (1969).
27 HORTON, B. T. Histaminic cephalgia resulting in production of acute duodenal ulcer. *J. Amer. med. Assoc.*, **122**, 59 (1943).
28 ——. Histaminic cephalgia (Horton's headache or syndrome). *Maryland med. J.*, **10**, 178–203 (1961).
29 JACOBSON, L. B. Cluster headache: a rare cause of bradycardia. *Headache*, **8**, 159–61 (1969).
30 KIRSCH, R. E., SAMET, P., KUGEL, V., and AXELROD, S. Electrocardiographic changes during ocular surgery and their prevention by retrobulbar injection. *Arch. Ophthal.* (*Chicago*), **58**, 348–56 (1957).

31 KUDROW, L. Prevalence of migraine, peptic ulcer, coronary heart disease and hypertension in cluster headache. *Headache*, **16**, 66–9 (1976).

32 KUNKLE, E. C. and ANDERSON, W. B. Dual mechanism of eye signs of headache in cluster pattern. *Trans. Amer. Neurol. Assoc.*, **85**, 75–9 (1960).

33 ——, PFEIFFER, J. B. JR., WILHOIT, W. M., and HAMRICK, L. W. JR. Recurrent brief headache in 'cluster' pattern. *Trans. Amer. Neurol. Assoc.*, **77**, 240–3 (1952).

34 LANCE, J. W. *Mechanism and management of headache* (3rd edn.). Butterworths, London (1978).

35 —— and ANTHONY, M. Migrainous neuralgia or cluster headache? *J. neurol. Sci.*, **13**, 401 (1971).

36 LENNOX, W. G. Science and seizures. In *New light on epilepsy and migraine* (1st edn.) Harper and Brothers, New York (1941).

37 LOVSHIN, L. L. Clinical caprices of histaminic cephalgia. *Headache*, **1**, 7–10 (1961).

38 NIEMAN, E. A. and HURWITZ, L. J. Ocular sympathetic palsy in periodic migrainous neuralgia. *J. Neurol. Neurosurg. Psychiat.*, **24**, 369–73 (1961).

39 OLESEN, J. Cluster headache associated with primary hyperlipidemia. *Acta Neurol. Scand.*, **56**, 461–4 (1977).

40 PALM, E. and STRÖMBLAD, R. Respiratory and circulatory responses to manipulations of the eye. *Acta Ophthal.* (Copenhagen), **32**, 615–29 (1954).

41 ROSENTHAL, M. *Diseases of the nervous system*, Vol. 2, pp. 254–6. William Wood, New York (1979).

42 SCHÉLE, R., AHLBORG, B., and EKBOM, K. Physical characteristics and allergic history in young men with migraine and other headaches. *Headache*, **18**, 80–6 (1978).

43 SHILLER, F. Prophylactic and other treatment for 'histaminic cluster', or 'limited' variant of migraine. *J. Amer. med. Assoc.*, **173**, 1907–11 (1960).

44 STEIN, C. Hereditary factors in epilepsy. *Amer. J. Psychiat.*, **12**, 989–1037 (1933).

45 SYMONDS, C. A particular variety of headache. *Brain*, **79**, 217–32 (1956).

46 Trends in cancer incidence. *Stat. Bull. Metropol. Life Ins. Co.*, **56**, 2–5 (Oct. 1975).

47 WATERS, W. E. and O'CONNOR, P. J. The clinical validation of a headache questionnaire. In *Background to migraine*, p. 1, 3rd British Migraine Symposium, Heinemann, London (1970).

6 Differential diagnosis

The diagnosis of cluster headache presents few difficulties. Periodicity and activity of the patient during attacks are pathognomonic features of this condition. The duration, location, and frequency of attacks and associated symptoms, are also quite constant from patient to patient. Headaches arising from other disorders, however, share one or more features of cluster headache. These include: temporal arteritis, pheochromocytoma, Raeder's syndrome, and trigeminal neuralgia. A description of these disorders and differentiation from cluster headache is presented in this chapter.

Table 6.1   Primary and secondary headache disorders

I. Primary	II. Secondary
A. Vascular	*A. Systemic disorders*
1. Migraine	1. Mechanisms
a Common, classical	a Vasodilatation
(1) Menstrual	(1) PGE synthesis
(2) Hormonal	(2) Cerebral hypoxia
(3) Menopausal	(3) Cerebral hypoglycaemia
(4) Tyramine	(4) Haemodynamic change
b Ophthalmic	b Traction
c Ophthalmoplegic	(1) Cerebral oedema
d Hemiplegic	c Vasculitis
e Basilar artery	*B. Intracranial disorders*
f Equivalents	1. Infection
2. Cluster	a Encephalitis
a Episodic	b Meningitis
b Chronic	c Abcess
(1) Primary	2. Tumour
(2) Secondary	3. Subdural
B. Muscle contraction	a Acute
1. Acute	b Chronic
2. Chronic	4. Acute bleeding
3. Post-traumatic	5. A-V anomaly
4. Conversion?	6. Ventricular obstruction
C. Nueralgias	
1. Trigeminal	
2. Atypical facial	
3. Post-herpatic	
4. Glossopharyngeal	
5. Superior laryngeal	
6. Eagle's syndrome	

Other primary headache disorders, such as migraine, combination headache, acute and chronic scalp muscle contraction headache, post-traumatic cephalgia, and conversion cephalgia, will be described in somewhat greater detail. The mechanisms and clinical features of headache secondary to systemic or intracranial disease is also included.

A classification of primary and secondary headache disorders is outlined in Table 6.1. Vascular headache, including migraine and its variants, cluster headache, muscle-contraction-type headaches and neuralgias, are all considered under primary headache disorders. Secondary headache disorders include systemic or intracranial diseases, where headache is a symptom.

Secondary headache disorders

Certain systemic diseases may cause alterations in cerebral blood concentrations of oxygen, carbon dioxide, and glucose to produce changes in cerebral blood-flow. Thus the major mechanism of headache associated with systemic disease, has an intracranial site and involves cerebrovascular dilatation. Distended cerebral arteries stimulate sensory end organs in the vessel wall, and cause focal oedema and pain. Cerebral oedema, with or without increased intracranial pressure, has also been shown to cause pain by traction or displacement of venous sinus structures and other pain-sensitive structures[15] (Table 6.2).

Cerebral vascular dilatation is the most common cause of systemic headache, and generally the result of pyrexia and infection.[45] The role of prostaglandins, as significant agents in pain production, has been described. More specifically, prostaglandin E has been reported by Ferreira[20] to cause intense pain and hyperalgesia of longer duration than that produced by histamine or bradykinin. Prostaglandins are also potent pyrogens. Its synthesis is inhibited by aspirin and other anti-inflammatory agents.[66] Furthermore, prostaglandins E and A directly dilate cerebral arteries.[44] It seems likely that these lipids, which are activated during infection, may be responsible for the headache associated with pyrexia and infection.

A decrease in cerebral oxygen content or, to a greater extent, increase in carbon dioxide tension, causes profound cerebrovascular dilatation.[74] Severe hypoxic states where venous oxygen saturation is 30 per cent or less produce unconsciousness and electroencephalo-

Table 6.2 Mechanisms of headache associated with systemic disease

Mechanism	Provoking condition or agent	Systemic state, disease

Cerebrovascular dilatation	Not yet defined (Prostaglandins?)	Pyrexia and infection
		  viraemia, bacteraemia
		  rickettsial disease

	Cerebral hypoxaemia	Anaemia
		  Deficiency states, blood loss
		  Myelophthisis
		  Haemolytic anaemias
		Polycythaemia
		  Chronic pulmonary disease
		  Congenital heart disease
		  Altitude sickness
		Toxic haemoglobinopathy
		  Carboxyhaemoglobinaemia
		  Methaemoglobinaemia
		  Sulphaemoglobinaemia
		Circulatory failure
		  Orthostatic hypotension
		  Cardiac arrest
		  Pulmonary artery obstruction

	Cerebral Hypoglycaemia	Systemic hypoglycaemia
		  Hyperinsulinism
		  Reactive hypoglycaemia
		  Hypothyroidism
		  Hypopituitarism
		  Addison's disease

	Haemodynamic changes	Hypertension
		  Essential hypertension
		  Acute (excitement)
		    hypertension
		  Pheochromocytoma

Traction on intracranial structures	Cerebral oedema	Hypertensive encephalopathy
		  eclampsia, benign
		  intracranial
		  hypertension, metastasis,
		  chronic renal diseases,
		  acute glomerulonephritis,
		  hepatic disease

graphic changes.[41] Cerebral hypoxaemia is associated with a wide range of disorders. These commonly include: anaemia, polycythaemia, congenital heart disease, haemoglobinopathy, or circulatory failure (Table 6.2).

Cerebral hypoglycaemia, as described by Brauch,[5] may cause headaches. Disorganization of electroencephalographic activity is observed with falling blood sugar levels. Actually, normal EEGs are rarely seen where blood sugar values are below 40–50 mg/ 100 ml.[52] Such changes are not unlike those seen with hypothyroidism, adrenal insufficiency, or hypopituitarism,[39] conditions frequently featuring hypoglycaemic headache.

Regarding haemodynamic changes, headache occurs with essential hypertension in about 50 per cent of the cases; however, elevation of blood-pressure solely is not sufficient to cause headache. A concomitant relaxation of the cerebral and cranial arteries is necessary.

There is evidence that cerebral oedema causes traction of intracranial pain-sensitive structures. Experimentally, an increase of cerebral spinal fluid pressure aggravated headache, whereas an intravenous infusion of manitol caused a decrease in intensity.[15] Cerebral oedema is notably present in hypertensive encephalopathy, a condition caused by several disease states (Table 6.2).

Metastatic tumours in the brain may also cause hypertensive encephalopathy. In order of greatest frequency, metastasis arises from the lung, thyroid, intestine, breast, stomach, kidney, adrenal, skin, and prostate.[1] In a series of 72 patients with primary brain tumours studied by Kunkle, Ray, and Wolff,[37] headache was a common complaint in 90 per cent of cases and was localized over the tumour site in one-third.

Benign intracranial hypertension (pseudotumour cerebri) is a syndrome characterized by increased intracranial pressure. Although intracranial disease is not demonstrable and the aetiology remains unknown, this syndrome has been associated with menstrual dysfunction, vitamin-A intoxication, cortical steroid therapy, hypoparathyroidism, hypoadrenalism, and tetracycline administration. The course appears to be self-limiting, and complications are uncommon.[15]

Characteristics of systemic headache (Table 6.3)

Headaches due to pheochromocytoma or temporal arteritis are excluded from this section. These conditions will be described later.

Headaches arising from fever or infection are often described as moderate to severe in intensity, throbbing in character, and associated with malaise and anorexia. Such headaches usually occur daily, often associated with temperature peaks. They may be constant in

Table 6.3 Characteristics of headache secondary to systemic conditions

Disease or condition	Timing related to	Frequency	Duration	Location	Intensity	Character	Associated signs and symptoms
Fever, infection	No consistent pattern	Usually daily	Intermittent or constant	Occipital, generalized bitemporal	Moderate to severe	Throbbing	Malaise, anorexia
Anaemia, polycythaemia, toxicity	Acute change	Usually daily	Hours to days	Occipital, or generalized	Dull if chronic, severe if acute	Throbbing	Related to cause
Hypoglycaemia	Post-exertional, Pre-prandial, insulin use	Almost daily	Minutes to hours	Generalized	Dull to moderate	Slight or non-throbbing	Sweating, confusion, restlessness
Essential hypertension	Morning, often awakening	Almost daily	Hours to constant	Occipital or generalized	Dull to moderate, increased in supine position	Throbbing at onset	Elevated B.P.
Hypertensive encephalopathy	No consistent pattern	Daily	Persistent	Generalized	Moderate to severe	Non-throbbing	Hypertension, azotaemia retinal haemorrhage
Cluster headache	Occurs with regularity, often awakens from sleep	1–3/day	30–90 min	Unilateral oculo-front. temporal	Excruciating	Non-throbbing boring	Unilateral lacrimation, rhinorrhoea injection, partial Horner's, cannot lie down

duration, or intermittent, generally located bilaterally, over the temple or occipital region.

Headaches arising from anaemia, polycythaemia, or toxicity are generally chronic. Such headaches may last hours to weeks. It is usually described as having an occipital or generalized location, being of dull intensity, and throbbing.

Hypoglycaemic headaches may occur as a result of hyperinsulinaemia or reactive hypoglycaemia. Otherwise, attacks may occur following exertion or prolonged periods of fasting. Attacks occur almost daily, last minutes to hours in duration, and are generalized in location. Intensity of pain is described as dull to moderate, and having a slight or non-throbbing component. Characteristic signs and symptoms of hypoglycaemic headache include restlessness, confusion, and profuse sweating.

Hypertensive headaches generally occur in the morning, often after awakening, on a daily basis. They are generally occipital in location, or generalized. Most often, the attacks persist only until the patient has been ambulatory for approximately one hour, but in a few cases, may remain constant. The headache is described as dull to moderate in intensity, and may increase in the supine position. Although headaches resulting from hypertensive encephalopathy have no consistent pattern, they are generally persistent, generalized in location, moderate to severe in intensity, and non-throbbing in character. Hypertension, azotaemia, and retinal haemorrhage are common findings in this condition.

The primary headache disorders

The five primary headache disorders described in this section are: migraine, two varieties of scalp muscle contraction headache, posttraumatic headache, and conversion cephalgia. Although some of these do not resemble cluster headache, they are included for completeness.

Migraine

Migraine is a physiological condition having headache as the outstanding clinical feature—as opposed to the earlier described headaches in which the headache symptom is secondary to a pathological process.

Approximately 25 per cent of women and 10 per cent of men have migraine.[70] Numerous reports have suggested that it is a genetic disorder affecting the vasomotor system.[3, 48] Goodell, Lewontin, and Wolff[22] concluded that the associated gene is probably an autosomal dominant, having an 80 per cent penetrance. In one study of monozygotic and dizygotic twin populations, however, significant concordance for migraine was lacking.[75]

Vasomotor instability leads to an increased reactivity of arteries under certain conditions, whereby patients often complain of cold hands and feet in the presence of only minimal stress. This tendency of peripheral vasoconstriction has been documented.[46]

The migraine attack has three phases.[11] The first is characterized by diminished cerebral vascular flow resulting in ischaemic cellular changes. If the occipital lobes are affected, a visual aura is experienced and may last from 10 to 30 minutes in duration. Scotomata begins with a pericentral field defect and migrates peripherally until it exits from the visual field.

The second stage is heralded by pain, mediated through extracranial vasodilatation. During this phase, cerebral blood-flow is also increased. The scalp arteries and perivascular tissue marks the third phase.

Classical migraine. Although typical in presentation, classical migraine is only one-tenth as common as ordinary (common) migraine. *Common migraine* is the most frequently occurring primary headache disorder. In contrast to other types, an obvious prodrome is not experienced. The headache phase, however, is otherwise similar and headache frequency is generally greater in this group, when compared to classical migraine.

Ophthalmic migraine has an incidence quite similar to that of classical migraine. Actually, ophthalmic migraine can be characterized as a classical migraine without the occurrence of a pain phase. Patients with ophthalmic migraine generally experience their scotomatous attacks infrequently, or on occasion, in bursts of two to three a week for short periods.

Hemiplegic migraine occurs quite infrequently and resembles classical migraine plus these added characteristics: unilateral extremity and facial numbness, weakness, and paraesthesias usually associated with dysphasia. This condition is strongly familial as first noted by Clark[9] as early as 1910 and as reviewed by Whitty[72] in 1953.

Ophthalmoplegic migraine was first described by Saundby[55] in 1882. It most often begins in early childhood and may recur throughout one's lifetime. Third-nerve paresis often occurs three to five days following onset of headache, and may last for as long as two to three months. Friedman, Harter, and Merritt[21] reported that of eight patients with ophthalmoplegic migraine, in a population of 5000 migraine patients, only one had involvement of both the third and fourth cranial nerves; and in another, permanent but partial damage of the oculomotor nerve resulted.

Basilar artery migraine is a rare form of migraine. It was first defined by Bickerstaff[4] in 1961. It most frequently affects young girls. Vertigo, ataxia, dysarthria, and tinnitis may be experienced following, or associated with, the pre-headache visual aura. In approximately 30 per cent of cases, syncopy may result, especially in young women, and last as long as 30 minutes. Following this period, as in classical migraine, the headache phase begins. It is believed that the cerebellar symptoms, that characterize this disorder, are due to involvement of the basilar-vertebral arteries.

Provoking factors. The increased frequency of migraine attacks among oral contraceptive users is well established.[23, 73] The cyclic use of moderately high doses of oestrogen preparations for replacement or supplemental therapy has been shown to increase migraine frequency.[36] In a recent study of 239 women with migraine, frequency of attacks was found to be significantly greater among oral contraceptive users (60 women), when compared to a group of women who were receiving oestrogen replacement or supplementation therapy (87 women), or to 92 women not using hormones. Moreover, upon discontinuance of oral contraceptives in the first group, and following reduction and 'decycling' of oestrogen in the second group, headache frequencies decreased by 70 and 80 per cent, respectively.[36]

Somerville[62] concluded that prolonged elevated levels of plasma oestrogen may prime cranial blood vessels, resulting in vasodilatation and headache, upon withdrawal. This may explain why, in the absence of extrinsic oestrogen use, attacks occur in association with menstruation. It may also account for the high incidence of migraine in women, generally. In this regard, it has been reported that although the female-to-male ratio of migraine in childhood is 1 : 1,[32] following menarche, it changes to favour women 2 : 1.[70] In headache clinics this latter ratio is closer to 4 : 1, or greater.

Numerous factors have been reported to induce acute migraine attacks. In an effort to identify these factors and establish their frequency of migraine induction, 400 patients at the California Medical Clinic for Headache were followed over a six-month period. In order of greatest frequency, the factors involved were: extrinsic oestrogen use; premenstrual and menstrual times; anticipatory anxiety; vacation periods; alcohol; weekends; post-crisis events; and chocolate. There was no significant influence of cigarette smoking, smog, weather change, season, ingestion of monosodium glutamate, sodium nitrate, or foods containing tyramine.[34] Ryan[53] and Shaw, Johnson, and Keogh[57] have also reported negative results regarding tyramine induction in migraine. This is in disagreement with the original studies of Hanington[24] published in 1967.

Another major factor in migraine induction appears to be stress, either resulting from anticipation, anxiety, or arising from bio-chemical changes related to adaptation effort. Clearly, migraine sufferers experience headache as a result of environmental change that may involve moving, job changes, and even vacations and week-ends. Vacations and week-ends are generally unstructured and may tax the adaptive abilities of rigid, intolerant, perfectionistic individuals. For these reasons, migraine may well be considered a maladaptation syndrome affecting psychological, biochemical, and vasomotor functions.

Biochemical changes. Specific biochemical events have been identi-fied in association with migraine and involve histamine, platelet serotonin, kinins, intrinsic heparin, monoamine oxidase (MAO), gamma-aminobutyric acid (GABA), prostaglandins, and tyramine. In 1961, Sicuteri, Testi, and Anselmi[58] found that the urinary turn-over rate of 5-hydroxy-indoleacetic acid, the major catabolic product of serotonin, was increased during the migraine attack. In 1967, Anthony, Hinterberger, and Lance[2] demonstrated that levels of platelet serotonin were elevated during the pre-headache phase and were decreased during the headache period.

During attacks, Thonnard-Neumann[65] observed an increased basophilic heparin level. This observation may be relevant since heparin affects platelet integrity.

During the migraine attack, alteration in neurotransmitter metabo-lism was inferred by the findings of Welch and associates.[71] They were able to demonstrate the presence of GABA in the spinal fluid of one group of patients with acute migraine, and in another group with cerebral vascular disease and ischaemia. Control groups, con-sisting of non-migraine headache sufferers and migraine sufferers in remission, showed no elevation of cerebral spinal fluid GABA levels.[71]

Other biochemical characteristics of migraine include: MAO deficiency and phenylethylamine oxidizing defects, as reported by Sandler, Youdim, and Hanington;[54] prostaglandin activity, as described by Carlson;[7] and the elicitation of histamine[61] and kinin increases.[8]

As noted earlier, oestrogen changes, stress, and dietary factors may precipitate a headache attack in genetically predisposed individuals. It is believed that these factors may induce platelet aggregability, as first reported by Kalendovsky and Austin.[31] This allows for the construction of a reasonable schema of migraine pathogenesis, one that incorporates most of the biochemical changes mentioned above.

Induced platelet aggregation leads to serotonin release, causing cerebral vascular constriction responsible for the pre-headache stage of migraine. Circulating serotonin induces prostaglandin release from lung tissue, which is in part, responsible for the profound extracranial arterial dilatation of the headache phase. Breakdown of circulating serotonin allows for an unopposed vasodilatation, contributing to the sustained, painful period. To this scheme, Fanchamps[19] suggests an additional step; as the platelets release serotonin, mast cells liberate histamine and proteolytic enzymes. Histamine and serotonin increases capillary permeability while proteolytic enzymes act on plasmakininogen, producing plasmakinin. Transudation of this substance causes vascular and perivascular pain, and with the combined action of reduced serotonin levels, reduces the pain threshold.

The migraine attack. Attacks may be described in terms of periodicity, symptoms, and signs. Characteristically, attacks occur from one to three times each month, frequently associated with menstrual periods. Each attack may last from one to three days, with some variation. Pain develops slowly over a period of several hours. In 80 per cent of cases the headache is unilateral, involving the temporal artery region and extending over the hemicranial area. Often, the pain is described as throbbing and associated with nausea, vomiting, photophobia, and sonophobia. Not infrequently, strong odours are poorly tolerated during the headache phase. Paraesthesias, hot and cold sensations, orthostatic lightheadedness, and anorexia may also be experienced during these episodes (Table 6.4).

Table 6.4 Attack characteristics of primary headache disorders

Disorder	Timing of attacks	Frequency	Duration	Location	Intensity	Character	Associated signs and symptoms
Migraine	Often menstrual	1–2/month	1–3 days	Hemicranial	Moderately severe	Throbbing	Nausea, vomiting, anorexia fatigue, paresthesia (aura in classical type)
CSMC†	No pattern	—Constant—		Frontoccip. or generalized	Dull	Non-throbbing	Depression
Post-traumatic	No pattern	—Constant—		Frontoccip., occipital, or generalized	Moderate	Non-throbbing	Occupational incapacitation, neuroticism
Conversion	No pattern	—Constant—		Generalized	Severe	Non-throbbing	Occupational and social incapacitation, neuroticism
Cluster	Occurs with regularity often awakens from sleep	1–3/day	30–90 min	Unilateral fronto-temporal	Excruciating	Non-throbbing; boring	Unilateral lacrimation rhinorrhoea injection, partial Horner's, cannot lie down

† Chronic scalp muscle contraction.

Chronic scalp muscle contraction headache

Adequate data concerning the incidence of chronic scalp muscle contraction headache in the general population is lacking. In our own headache clinic, approximately 44 per cent of all patients have this type of headache. The most common form in which chronic scalp muscle contraction presents is in patients who also have migraine headaches. The occurrence of chronic scalp muscle contraction headache and migraine headache in the same patient is called 'combination headache'.

Pain mechanisms. In 1944, Elliott[18] reported that sustained muscle contraction, as evidenced by increased action potential change, is painful. Lewis[42] demonstrated that voluntary muscle contraction over a two-minute duration produced pain and often outlasted the contraction itself. According to Hinsey,[27] pain impulses are conveyed from terminal branches in the adipose and connective tissue of muscle to its afferent nerve fibres in the adventitia of small vessels. Simons, Day, Goodell, and Wolff[59] in a series of experiments described the vascular and myogenic changes associated with spontaneous and induced scalp muscle contraction pain. A summary of these findings was enumerated by Dalessio.[14] It was demonstrated that scalp muscle pain was indeed caused by muscle contraction and was accompanied by extracranial vasoconstriction. Vasoconstriction alone was ruled out as a source of pain; an observation recently verified by Rodbard.[50] He showed that in the absence of ischaemia, hypoxaemia, or lactic acidosis, contracting muscles released a catabolite capable of producing pain.

Patients with chronic scalp muscle contraction headache have been described as depressed, anxious, repressive, and dependent. Such were the findings of Martin[43] who had obtained MMPI evaluations on 50 such patients. So consistent was the finding of depression in Diamond's[16] series that he coined the term 'depression headache' to describe chronic scalp muscle contraction headache.

In 1976, the Zung Self-Rating Depression Scale Test (SDS)[76] was administered to 670 patients with chronic scalp muscle contraction headache at the California Medical Clinic for Headache. The mean index score was 53·2; 62·3 per cent scored above 50.[35] (An index score of over 50 is consistent with depression.)

Independently, Lance and Curran[38] and Diamond and Baltes[17] have reported that prophylactic tricyclic antidepressants were effec-

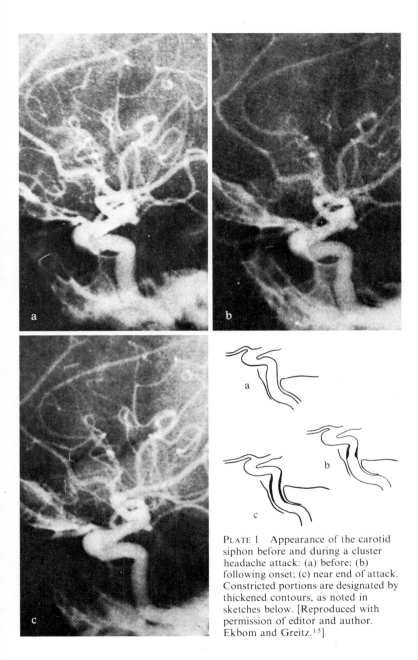

PLATE 1 Appearance of the carotid siphon before and during a cluster headache attack: (a) before; (b) following onset; (c) near end of attack. Constricted portions are designated by thickened contours, as noted in sketches below. [Reproduced with permission of editor and author. Ekbom and Greitz.[15]]

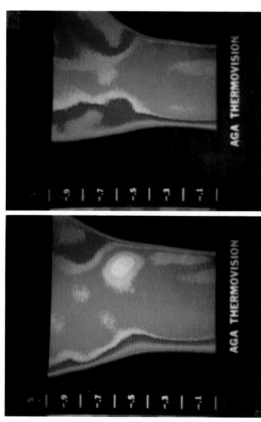

PLATE 2 Thermal view of the right wrist. (a) Area of maximal heat (yellow colour) corresponds to the distal segment of the radial artery; (b) following tourniquet occlusion of blood flow, arterial heat vanishes. [From Kudrow.[34]]

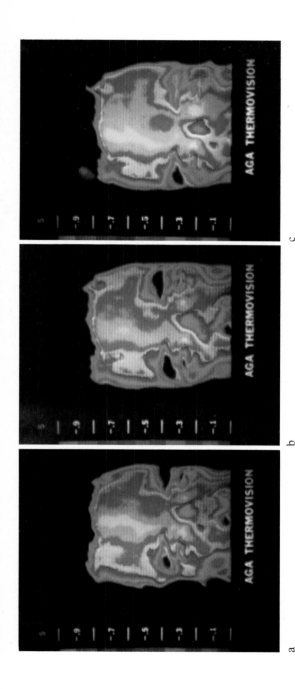

PLATE 3 Facial thermography of a patient with left-sided cluster headaches. Supraorbital arterial heat is asymmetric, greater on the right. Compression of the right temporal artery (a) causes increased heat over supraorbital artery, corresponding to augmentation of internal carotid artery flow; (b) shows the situation before arterial compression. Left temporal artery compression; (c) augments left internal carotid artery flow and increases flow to the right side via anastomosis of the frontal arteries. Each colour change represents 0·5 C difference. Order of colours from warmest to coolest are: yellow, gold, red, violet, dark blue, and light blue. [From Kudrow.[34]]

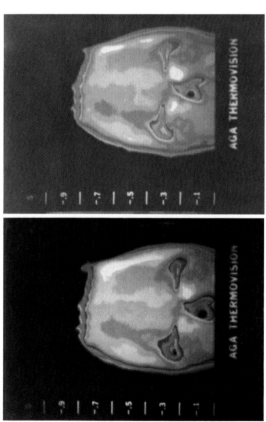

PLATE 4 Facial thermography of a right-sided cluster patient, obtained during an interim state. (a) Before compression; (b) following left (contralateral) temporal artery compression.

tive in chronic scalp muscle contraction headache. Dalessio[12,13] suggested that since tricyclics increase the availability of cerebral norepinephrine, as was shown by Schildkraut, Schanberg, Breese, and Kopin,[56] depletion of this amine may be responsible for this condition and its frequently associated depression.

Pain characteristics. Scalp muscle contraction headaches do not show temporal patterns. It is constantly present, generally located in frontal-occipital or occipital regions, or may be generalized. The intensity of pain is dull, mild, or annoying, and non-throbbing in character. As noted earlier, depression and hysteria are commonly associated findings (Table 6.4).

Post-traumatic headache

Chronic post-traumatic headache (P-T) is defined as a persistent or recurring headache, originating from an accident or injury. The disorder may arise from injury to the head, neck, or other anatomical structure; or may result from accidents in which no apparent injury had occurred. Moderate to severe head injury, followed by intractable headaches has been the subject of numerous studies. Walker and Jablon[69] reported an 80 per cent incidence of P-T, of many years duration, among 739 head-wounded veterans. In his retrospective study of 230 patients who had sustained cerebral contusions, Jacobson[30] also found that 80 per cent had chronic post-traumatic headache. Brenner, Friedman, Merritt, and Denny-Brown[6] noted an incidence of less than 50 per cent, among patients requiring hospitalization.

Simons and Wolff[60] developed a classification based on headache characteristics in their study of 63 post-traumatic patients, of whom 50 per cent had sustained severe head injury. They defined three types. Type 1 presented as having a pressure type pain, dull intensity, band-like in distribution, and tender to palpation. The presence of circumscribed tenderness, superimposed over a generalized, diffuse, dull pain, distinguished Type 2. The third type was characterized by paroxysmal, unilateral, severe and throbbing pain. Of their 63 patients, 70 per cent had Type 1, solely; 24 per cent, Type 2; and 6 per cent, Type 3. In Type 1 patients, they were able to demonstrate increased action potentials, recorded from scalp muscles, at or near the areas of head pain. Furthermore, changes in recorded muscle potentials corresponded to the changes in pain intensity. These findings have established a relationship of post-traumatic headache to chronic scalp muscle contraction headache.

Most post-traumatic headache patients seen in headache clinics, present with a history of mild head injury or no head injury. The headache characteristics are quite similar to those of chronic scalp muscle contraction headache and conversion cephalgia. In addition, chronic post-traumatic headaches that follow minimal injury are indistinguishable from those resulting from moderate or severe head injury, as described by other clinicians.[6, 60, 68] Also Jacobson[30] reported no significant difference in the incidence of chronic post-traumatic headache between minimally injured, and moderately to severely head-injured individuals.

Table 6.5 Frequency of abnormal test results and correlation to head injury in 29 patients with post-traumatic headache

Head injury	N	Reitan Psychophysiologic Battery				Depression Test (SDS)	
		Impairment index (> 0·4)		Dysphasia (> 1 symptom)		Mod-severe (> 60)	
		N	(per cent)	N	(per cent)	N	(per cent)
Mod–severe	12	7	58·3	7	58·3	5	41·7
Minor or none	17	8	47·1	7	41·2	5	29·4

Since post-traumatic patients are indistinguishable, in regard to the severity of injury, we undertook a study of 29 post-traumatic patients using a psychophysiological test battery, as developed by Reitan.[49] It includes a series of performance tests designed to measure the quality of function of specific cortical regions. An impairment index score of greater than 0·4 was considered evidence of cortical dysfunction. Similarly, more than one dysphasic symptom was considered evidence of abnormal cerebral function. Our results showed that approximately 50 per cent of both groups, the mildly injured and severely injured, had scored in the impairment range. We concluded that there is no correlation between post-traumatic headache and extent of injury, as measured by this psychophysiological test battery (Table 6.5). Our data suggested that cortical impairment was not a result of physical injury in these cases, but rather the consequence of the traumatic experience.[33]

Headache characteristics. The largest percentage of patients with post-traumatic headaches described the pain as rather constant or persistent, having no pattern in relation to time or day. Pain is often generalized or located across the fronto-occipital or occipital areas, and is dull to moderate in intensity. This most common type is generally non-throbbing. Many of these patients will complain of a secondary vascular component headache, often unilateral in location, moderate to severe in intensity, and throbbing in character; this may be experienced several times a week. In some migraine patients who develop post-traumatic headache, the attack profile may be indistinguishable from that of migraine headache. Patients with post-traumatic headache are often occupationally incapacitated (Table 6.4).

Conversion cephalgia

The term 'conversion cephalgia' derives from 'conversion hysteria', a type of hysterical neurosis. Both conditions are marked by related or similar psychological defence mechanisms and emotional symptoms, such as denial in the one, and repression in the other. Both are also characterized by *belle indifférence*.

The somatic manifestations of the two, however, are quite dissimilar. In hysterical neurosis, such symptoms characteristically appear and disappear suddenly in response to stressful situations involving the voluntary, rather than the autonomic nervous system. Also, hysterical neurosis is amenable to psychotherapy. The somatic profile of conversion cephalgia is, however, indistinguishable from that associated with 'psychophysiological disorders'. Therefore, conversion cephalgia is a mixed entity, having both psychosomatic and neurotic components.

Characteristics. Patients having conversion cephalgia are generally somewhat older than those having other primary headache disorders. Typically, the patient has a history of headache of several years duration. The headache is described as being constant, and having no temporal patterns. Similar to post-traumatic cephalgia, its location is often occipital, frontal-occipital or generalized. It is a non-throbbing headache and characteristically described as having a severe intensity. Despite their description of incapacitating pain, patients reveal no apparent evidence of discomfort, exhibiting an apathetic facies (*belle indifférence*). Curiously, the sufferer of either sex is accompanied by her spouse when seeking medical consultation. The spouse appears excessively parental and doting in his behaviour.

He may portray his role as that of the 'official back-rubber', medication controller, cook, and housekeeper.

This condition is also characterized by the patient's excessive use of analgesics, narcotic, or non-narcotics; barbiturates for sleep and tranquillizers are commonly used. This condition is markedly resistant to most forms of therapy. Despite the presence of significant depression, tricyclic antidepressants are usually ineffective, while phenothiazines appear to aggravate the general emotional state. Moreover, muscle relaxants are of little benefit. It is likely that analgesics contribute to their drug dependency and may, in fact, be partly responsible for their emotional state. Antimigraine medication affords no relief and the results of outpatient psychotherapy are discouraging, associated with a high drop-out rate. Hence, the psychodynamics of this condition are poorly understood (Table 6.4).

Results of MMPI testing among patients having primary headache disorders. In spite of a preponderance of psychometric testing reported in the headache literature, psychopersonality structures of patients with primary headache disorders remain ill-defined. Specifically, reports concerning MMPI evaluations in headache appear to be inconsistent with clinical experience.

In an excellent review of psychological testing in headache, Harrison[25] stated that the MMPI is a major test relevant to levels of objective observation. In his review, he concluded that headache patients score above average on MMPI scales measuring neurotic anxiety.

Although this may be the case for headache patients in general, it may not be applicable to headache disorders, individually. Attempts to evaluate certain headache groups have had ambiguous results. For example, of the five MMPI studies reviewed by Harrison[25] only two defined migraine as a specific group. Henryk-Gutt and Rees[26] found no difference between migraine and control groups, using 'quick' MMPI tests. Conversely, Rogado, Harrison, and Graham[51] characterized the migraine group as neurotic, compared to controls.

It is unlikely that intrinsic deficiencies of the MMPI are responsible for this discrepancy since scoring values are standardized, and its reliability is generally respected. There is much less reliability, however, in headache diagnosis, especially concerning combination headache. Patients having migraine as their sole headache disorder may be quite different psychologically than those who have a combination of headache disorders. In fact, the latter situation is more frequently seen in headache clinics, as noted earlier.

As reported in 1978, Dr Bruce Sutkus and I, obtained and compared MMPI test results from specific headache groups, comprising six primary headache disorders.[33] Subjects from whom MMPIs were obtained were new out-patients of the California Medical Clinic for Headache seeking consultation for headache complaints. Excluded from the study were patients under 18 and over 70 years of age, foreign patients having language difficulties, and patients experiencing ergotamine rebound, or using birth control pills. In all cases, intracranial and systemic disease were ruled out as the cause of headache.

MMPI results from 255 patients were obtained over an allotted three-month collection period, limiting each diagnostic group to 32 women and 20 men. The reverse of this was true for the cluster headache category. Control groups consisted of 15 male and 15 female non-patient subjects of varying occupations and life-styles. Profile sheets were separated and classified by diagnostic category. Mean values for each MMPI scale included the k value computation. All data was computerized and subjected to statistical analysis with the assistance of the Health Sciences Computing Facility, at UCLA. Comparisons of 13 scales (3 validity and 10 clinical) from male and female diagnostic categories, were subjected to f (variance) and t tests, providing probability values of significance.

Our results showed that scores from patients with migraine were almost indistinguishable from those with cluster headache. Similarly, scalp muscle contraction headache patients and patients with combination headache, scored alike. Furthermore, patients with post-traumatic headache were almost indistinguishable from those with conversion cephalgia.[33] These results would indicate that psychologically, or in terms of personality characteristics, there may be an aetiological relationship between these paired headache disorders.

Scales 1, 2, and 3, reflecting hypochondriasis, depression, and hysteria, respectively, are generally considered measures of neuroses when elevated above a t score level of 65.[40] Such was the case for all headache groups with the exception of either migraine or cluster, of either sex (Tables 6.6 and 6.7).[33]

The oft-reported perfectionistic, rigid, obsessive-compulsive traits of the migraineur was not confirmed by the study. Migraine and cluster males were not characterized by the conversion 'v' pattern. Hence, evidence of neuroticism associated with either migraine or

Table 6.6 MMPI mean scale scores in female headache categories

Scales	Controls	Headache categories					
		Migraine	Cluster	CSMC†	Combination	P-T‡	Conversion
L	3·0	3·7	3·6	3·6	3·6	4·2	3·3
F	4·9	5·4	5·9	7·3	5·8	8·4	8·3
K	15·7	13·3	14·0	12·8	15·3	14·7	13·3
1	11·9	16·2	15·1	19·9**	19·6**	22·5***	22·8***
2	18·3	23·1	23·0	27·5***	26·0**	29·4***	28·7***
3	21·1	23·9	23·9	26·3*	29·4**	31·8***	32·1***
4	21·3	20·9	22·5	24·2	24·0	27·8**	25·1
5	27·8	26·8	26·6	25·6	28·1	26·3	27·1
6	8·0	9·6	10·1	9·9	11·4	12·1	11·2
7	24·1	28·4	26·8	29·5	31·5	32·8**	33·8**
8	23·4	26·0	24·0	29·9	28·6	33·8**	34·1**
9	20·3	19·6	19·7	19·1	20·5	21·1	21·2
10	23·9	29·8	27·9	32·2	30·7	30·2	30·9

† CSMC = chronic scalp muscle contraction. t scores: * 65–9; ** 70–4; *** > 74.
‡ P-T = post-traumatic cephalgia.

Table 6.7 MMPI mean scale scores in male headache categories

Scales	Controls	Headache categories					
		Migraine	Cluster	CSMC†	Combination	P-T‡	Conversion
L	3·0	3·7	4·1	4·3	3·5	4·6	4·6
F	4·2	4·7	7·0	6·2	6·6	6·6	9·0
K	16·8	14·6	13·8	13·4	12·2	13·3	13·7
1	12·3	18·4	17·8	21·5*	21·0*	23·7**	26·9***
2	20·3	23·7	23·8	27·7*	28·5*	27·4*	33·9***
3	20·7	27·0	25·6	30·3*	28·0*	31·8***	36·3***
4	20·5	22·4	23·6	24·0	23·4	24·3	26·7**
5	39·4	38·8	37·4	38·5	40·7	38·6	38·2
6	7·5	10·4	11·8	10·3	11·4	11·9	12·8
7	25·0	29·4	25·9	31·5	33·8	33·0	37·2*
8	25·7	26·7	25·9	29·0	30·2	32·4	38·0**
9	19·0	19·9	19·1	18·2	19·7	23·1	19·8
10	26·9	29·4	24·6	32·1	35·4	28·7	35·4

† CSMC = chronic scalp muscle contraction.
‡ P-T = post-traumatic cephalgia.

t scores: * 65–9; ** 70–4; *** > 74.

cluster was not found, differing widely from other reports.[51, 63] This disparity may relate to diagnostic specificity since, according to our findings, migraineurs contaminated with 'other headache components' are likely to have MMPI profiles consistent with neuroses. This is evidenced by the scores obtained from patients in the chronic scalp muscle contraction, combination, post-traumatic, and conversion groups. Scales 1, 2, and 3 in the chronic scalp muscle contraction and combination headache groups, have t score elevations between 65 and 74; t score elevations between 70 and 80, however, were seen in five or six scales (1, 2, 3, 4, 7, 8) from post-traumatic and conversion headache groups (Tables 6.6 and 6.7).[33]

These findings suggested a continuum of psychopathology, beginning with migraine and cluster (as containing little or none) through combination and scalp muscle contraction headache, to post-traumatic and conversion cephalgia, the latter reflecting the most severe pathology.

Conditions in which headaches resemble cluster headache

The headaches associated with certain disorders, other than primary headache disorders, have some characteristics resembling cluster headache. These include trigeminal neuralgia, pheochromocytoma, temporal arteritis, and Raeder's paratrigeminal syndrome.

Trigeminal neuralgia

Trigeminal neuralgia occurs with equal frequency in men and women and generally occurs in older age groups. Dalessio[10] proposed that tic douloureaux is a disease state of relative disordered cortical inhibition. He stated that the trigger zones of tic douloureaux may represent peripheral manifestations of a hyperexcitable area of the nervous system, as though a portion of the sensory input through a small area of the trigeminal nerve was operating in a 'strychninized' circuit, lacking inhibition. Strychnine, he notes, does not produce excitation from direct synaptic stimulation, but rather, by a selectively blocking inhibition. When such inhibition is blocked, neuronal activity is enhanced, and sensory stimuli will induce exaggerated reflex effects. Furthermore, strychnine does not excite neuronal systems lacking specific inhibitory fibres. Thus, autonomic ganglia are not stimulated by this substance. He further states that carbamazepine, a drug that is successfully used in tic douloureaux, is an antagonist to strychnine and will decrease the reactivity of trigger zones, at about the time it relieves the pain sequence of tic douloureaux. This strychnine model supports the hypothesis that carbamazepine acts as if it were increasing post-synaptic inhibition of sensory input in the trigeminal circuit.[10]

Characteristics. The pain of trigeminal neuralgia is characterized as severe, razor-sharp, electric-like, or cutting. It is precipitated by the touching of trigger zones on the face, ipsilaterally. These zones are most commonly found in an area around the nasolabial folds, but may occur anywhere from the chin to the forehead. Activation of the trigger site may result from the slightest touch, including even a gentle breeze across the face. Most frequently, the act of eating, chewing, or shaving triggers the attack.

The attack begins with a slight sensation of gentle jabbing over the involved site and is followed by a session of lightning tics that last for seconds to minutes. The attack may begin abruptly without warning sensations. An important observation differentiating tic douloureaux from cluster headache is that in the former, attacks are not likely to occur in the middle of the night, awakening the patient from sleep (Table 6.8).

Raeder's paratrigeminal syndrome

In 1924, based on observations in six patients, Raeder first reported the disorder presently known as a Raeder's paratrigeminal syndrome. The primary manifestations were unilateral head pain, ptosis and miosis without anhidrosis, thereby distinguishing it from Horner's syndrome. Raeder[47] suggested that the pathogenesis of this disorder involved the oculosympathetic nerve in the region of the trigeminal ganglion, due to either trauma, or disease.[47]

Following a review of Raeder's publications and all other reports regarding this syndrome, Vijayan and Watson[67] concluded that the location of the lesion was in the pericarotid, rather than the paratrigeminal region. They attempted to elucidate the actual route of the oculosympathetic fibres, from the spinal cord to the eye, using various clinical and experimental observations from the literature; data from six of their own cases, and, by dissection of cadaver material, to prove their hypothesis. In all of their cases, the sweat test showed ipsilateral supraorbital anhidrosis, which they admit, although positive, was clinically difficult to delineate.[67]

Pain characteristics. The pain of Raeder's syndrome is generally

Table 6.8 Characteristics of headache attacks which resemble cluster

Conditions resembling cluster	Timing of attacks	Frequency	Duration	Location	Intensity	Character	Associated signs and symptoms
Trigeminal neuralgia	No pattern	Several per day	Seconds to minutes	Unilateral, 5th nerve distribution	Severe	Electric, lancinating, non-throbbing	Trigger zones on face
Temporal arteritis	No pattern	Persistent		Unilateral, temporal	Severe	Burning, throbbing, non-throbbing	Chewing claudication, tender and tortuous temporal artery, elevated ESR, polymyalgia
Pheochromocytoma	Mornings, often on awakening	Daily to monthly	Less than one hour	Bilateral, occipital	Severe in supine position	Throbbing	Sweating, pallor, tachycardia with rise in blood-pressure
Raeder's syndrome	Often awakens from sleep	Persistent	Persistent	Unilateral, supraocular	Severe	Burning, throbbing, non-throbbing	Partial Horner's syndrome
Cluster	Occurs with regularity, often awakens from sleep	1–3/day	30–90 min	Unilateral, oculo-front. temporal	Excruciating	Non-throbbing, boring	Unilateral lacrimation, rhinorrhoea, injection, partial Horner's, cannot lie down

persistent and may last from weeks to months. During the first couple of weeks the patient is likely to be awakened in the middle of the night with severe, unilateral, supraorbital pain of a burning, throbbing, or non-throbbing character. Early in the course, the severe pain may cease towards the afternoon. Later in the course, the pain is less severe, but continuous. As noted earlier, drooping of the ipsilateral eyelid associated with miosis, are associated features. It would appear that if a small area of anhidrosis is present it would probably not be observed clinically and may be difficult to elucidate, using this sweat test. This disorder has several features easily confused with cluster headache, such as, partial Horner's syndrome, ipsilateral severe and burning supraorbital pain and may awaken the patient in the middle of the night. Unlike cluster headache, however, the pain's duration is constant (Table 6.8).

Temporal arteritis

In 1932, Horton, Magath, and Brown[28] first described temporal arteritis. In a recent epidemiologic, clinical, and pathologic study, Huston, Hunder, Lie, Kennedy, and Elveback[29] reported the over-all incidence of temporal arteritis as, $2 \cdot 4/100\,000$ total population.

Clearly, temporal arteritis affects older age groups. Arteries are affected, in highest to lowest order of frequency as follows: superficial temporal, vertebral, ophthalmic, posterior ciliac, internal carotid, external carotid, and central retinal arteries. Although the disease is self-limiting, if untreated, it often results in blindness. In approximately 50 per cent of the cases, a non-specific aching or stiffness of the neck, shoulders, or hip girdle precede the onset of head pain by several months (polymyalgia rheumatica). The head pain is described as persistent, waxing and waning throughout the day, unilateral in location, directly related to the superficial temporal artery. It is severe, burning, and throbbing in the early course of the disease, and non-throbbing later. Characteristically, the superficial temporal artery is tender to palpation and reveals a marked firmness and tortuousity. Claudication upon chewing is frequently experienced as an associated feature. The sedimentation rate is generally elevated quite markedly (Table 6.8). The finding of giant cells on temporal artery biopsies are diagnostic of this condition. Based on their survey, Huston *et al.* [29] estimated that clinically active temporal arteritis lasts approximately one year, assuming that the patients had been treated with cortical steroids as long as needed.

Pheochromocytoma

The paroxysmal hypertensive episode seen in pheochromocytoma is associated with catecholamine release followed by head pain, pallor, tachycardia, and profuse sweating. Thomas, Rooke, and Kvale[64] thoroughly described the headache of pheochromocytoma. They found that of 100 patients, 80 experienced headache as an outstanding symptom. The pain was described as paroxysmal, rapid in onset, and severe; often awakening the patient during early morning hours and commonly induced during exertion. The headaches were characterized as throbbing, almost always bilateral and occipital, suboccipital or fronto-occipital, in location. Coughing, sneezing, bending, and straining, aggravated the pain. Attacks had occurred with a daily to monthly frequency and generally lasted less than one hour (Table 6.8).

References

1 ANDERSON, A. *Pathology.* (3rd edn.) The C. V. Mosby Co., St Louis, Missouri (1957).
2 ANTHONY, M., HINTERBERGER, H., and LANCE, J. W. Plasma serotonin in migraine and stress. *Arch. Neurol.* (*Chicago*), 16, 544–52 (1967).
3 BAROLIN, G. S. and SPERLICH, D. Migraine Familien. *Fortsch. Neurol. Psychiat.*, 37, 521–54 (1969).
4 BICKERSTAFF, E. R. Basilar artery migraine. *Lancet*, 1, 15–17 (1961).
5 BRAUCH, F. Hypoglycemic headache. *Dtsch. med. Wochenschr.*, 76, 828 (1951).
6 BRENNER, C., FRIEDMAN, A. P., MERRITT, H. H., and DENNY-BROWN, D. Post-traumatic headache. *J. Neurosurg*, 1, 379 (1944).
7 CARLSON, L. A. Metabolic and cardiovascular effects *in vivo* of prostaglandins. In *Prostaglandins* (ed. S. Bergstrom and B. Samuelson), pp. 123–61. Nobel Symposium 2, Interscience, New York (1967).
8 CHAPMAN, L. F., RAMOS, A. O., GOODELL, H., SILVERMAN, G., and WOLFF, H. G. Humoral agent implicated in vascular headache of the migraine type. *Arch. Neurol.* (*Chicago*), 3, 223–9 (1960).
9 CLARKE, J. M. On recurrent motor paralysis in migraine; with report of a family in which recurrent hemiplegia accompanied the attacks. *Brit. med. J.*, 1, 1534–8 (1910).
10 DALESSIO, D. J. A reappraisal of the trigger zones of tic douloureaux. *Headache*, 9, 73–6 (1969).
11 ———. Classification of headache. *Int. Ophthal. Clin.*, 10, 647–65 (1970).

12 ——. Chronic pain syndromes and disordered cortical inhibition: effects of tricyclic compounds. *Dis. nerv. Sys.*, **28**, 325 (1967).

13 ——. Some reflections on the etiologic role of depression in head pain. *Headache*, **8**, 28–31 (1968).

14 ——. *Wolff's headache and other head pain.* (3rd edn.), pp. 525–83. Oxford University Press, New York (1972).

15 ——. *Wolff's headache and other head pain,* (3rd edn.) Oxford University Press, New York (1972).

16 DIAMOND, S. Depression headaches. *Headache*, **4**, 255–8 (1964).

17 —— and BALTES, B. J. Chronic tension headache treated with amitriptyline—a double blind study. *Headache*, **11**, 110–16 (1971).

18 ELLIOTT, F. A. Tender muscles in sciatica. Electromyographic studies. *Lancet*, **1**, 47–9 (1944).

19 FANCHAMPS, A. The role of humoral mediators in migraine headache. *Can. J. neurol. Sci.*, **1**, 189–95 (1974).

20 FERREIRA, S. H. Prostaglandins, aspirin-like drugs and analgesia. *Nature (New Biol.)*, **240**, 200 (1972).

21 FRIEDMAN, A. P., HARTER, D. H., and MERRITT, H. H. Ophthalmoplegic migraine. *Arch. Neurol.*, **7**, 82–7 (1962).

22 GOODELL, H., LEWONTIN, R. and WOLFF, H. G. Familial occurrence of migraine headache. *Arch. neurol. Psychiat.*, **72**, 325–34 (1954).

23 GRANT, E. C. G. Relation between headaches from oral contraceptives and development of endometrial arterioles. *Brit. med. J.*, **3**, 402–5 (1968).

24 HANINGTON, E. Preliminary report on tyramine headache. *Brit. med. J.*, **2**, 550–1 (1967).

25 HARRISON, R. H. Psychological testing in headache: a review. *Headache*, **13**, 177–85 (1975).

26 HENRYK-GUTT, R. and REES, W. L. Psychological aspects of migraine. *J. psychosom. Res.*, **17**, 141–53 (1973).

27 Hinsey, J. C. Observations on the innervation of the blood vessels in skeletal muscle. *J. comp. Neurol.*, **47**, 23–65 (1928).

28 HORTON, B. T., MAGATH, T. B., and BROWN, G. E. An undescribed form of arteritis of the temporal vessels. *Proc. Staff Meet. Mayo. Clin.*, **7**, 700–1 (1932).

29 HUSTON, K. A., HUNDER, G. G., LIE, J. T., KENNEDY, B. A. and ELVEBACK, L. R. Temporal arteritis. A 25-year epidemiologic, clinical, and pathologic study. *Ann. intern. Med.*, **88**, 162–7 (1978).

30 JACOBSON, S. A. Mechanisms of the sequelae of minor craniocervical trauma. In *The late effects of head injury* (1st edn.) (ed. A. E. Calker, W. F. Caveness, and M. Critchley), pp. 33–45. Charles C. Thomas Springfield, Illinois. (1969).

31 KALENDOVSKY, Z. and AUSTIN, J. H. 'Complicated migraine', its association with increased platelet aggregability and abnormal plasma coagulation factors. *Headache*, **15**, 18–35 (1975).

32 KRUPP, G. R. and FRIEDMAN, A. P. Migraine in children. A report of fifty children. Read before the Section of Pediatrics, 101st Annual Session of AMA, Chicago (June 1950).

33 KUDROW, L. and SUTKUS, B. J. Chronic post-traumatic headache:

psychophysiological assessment of minimally injured patients. Presentation, 21st Annual Meeting of The American Association for the Study of Headache, Boston, Massachusetts (23 June 1979).

34 ——. Current aspects of migraine headache. *Psychosom.*, **19**, 48–57 (1978).

35 ——. Tension headache (scalp muscle contraction headache). In *Pathogenesis and treatment of headache* (ed. O. Appenzeller), pp. 81–91. Spectrum Publications Inc., New York (1976).

36 ——. The relationship of headache frequency to hormone use in migraine. *Headache*, **15**, 36–40 (1975).

37 KUNKLE, E. C., RAY, B. S., and WOLFF, H. G. Studies on headache: The mechanisms and significance of headaches associated with brain tumor. *Bull. NY Acad. Med.*, **18**, 400 (1942).

38 LANCE, J. W. and CURRAN, D. A. Treatment of chronic tension headache *Lancet*, **1**, 1236–9 (1964).

39 LANSING, R. W. and TRUNNELL, J. B. Electroencephalographic changes accompanying thyroid deficiency in man. *J. Clin. Endocrinol. Metab.*, **23**, 470–80 (1963).

40 LANYON, R. I. *A Handbook of MMPI group profiles*, pp. 6–7. University of Minnesota Press (1968).

41 LENNOX, W. G., GIBBS, F. A., and GIBBS, E. L. The relationship in man of cerebral activity to blood flow and to blood constituents. *J. Neurol. Neurosurg. Psychiat.*, **1**, 211–25 (1938).

42 LEWIS, T. Pain and tenderness in ischaemic muscle. In *Pain*, pp. 97–9. MacMillan, New York (1942).

43 MARTIN, M. J. Tension headache, a psychiatric study. *Headache*, **6**, 47–54 (1966).

44 NAKANO, J. Effects of prostaglandins on the coronary and peripheral circulations. *Proc. Soc. Exp. Biol. Med.*, **127**, 1160–3 (1938).

45 PICKERING, G. W. Experimental observations of headache. *Brit. med. J.*, **1**, 4087 (1939).

46 PRICE, K. P. and TURSKY, B. Vascular reactivity of migraineurs and nonmigraineurs: a comparison of responses to self-control procedures. *Headache*, **16**, 210–7 (1976).

47 RAEDER, J. G. 'Paratrigeminal' paralysis of oculo-pupillary sympathetic. *Brain*, **47**, 149–58 (1924).

48 REFSUM, S. Genetic aspects of migraine. In *Handbook of clinical neurology* (ed. P. J. Vinken and G. W. Bruyn), Vol. 5, Ch. 25. North-Holland Publishing Co., Amsterdam (1968).

49 REITAN, R. M. Assessment of brain-behaviour relationships. In *Advances in psychological assessment* (ed. P. McReynolds), Vol. 3, pp. 186–242. Josey-Bass Inc., San Francisco (1974).

50 RODBARD S. Pain associated with muscle contraction. *Headache*, **10**, 105–115 (1970).

51 ROGADO, A., HARRISON, R. H., and GRAHAM, J. R. Personality profiles in cluster headache, migraine and normal controls. Read at 10th International Congress of World Federation of Neurology (Sept. 1973).

52 ROSS, I. S., and LOESER, L. H. Electroencephalographic findings in

essential hypoglycemia. *Electroencephal. clin. Neurophysiol.*, **3**, 33–42 (1940).
53 RYAN, R. E. SR. A clinical study of tyramine as an etiological factor in migraine. *Headache*, **14**, 43–8 (1974).
54 SANDLER, M., YOUDIM, M. B. H., and HANINGTON, E. A phenylethylamine oxidizing defect in migraine. *Nature*, **250**, 335–41 (1974).
55 SAUNDBY, R. A case of megrim, with paralysis of the third nerve. *Lancet*, **2**, 345–6 (1882).
56 SCHILDKRAUT, J. J., SCHANBERG, S. M., BREESE, G. R., and KOPIN, I. J. Norepinephrine metabolism and drugs used in the affective disorders: a possible mechanism of action. *Amer. J. Psychiat.*, **124**, 54–62 (1967).
57 SHAW, S. W. J., JOHNSON, R. H., and KEOGH, H. J. Oral tyramine in dietary migraine sufferers. Read before the Migraine Trust, International Symposium, London (Sept. 1976).
58 SICUTERI, F., TESTI, A., and ANSELMI, B. Biochemical investigation in headache: increase in the hydroxyindoleacetic acid excretion during migraine attacks. *Int. Arch. Allerg.*, **19**, 55–8 (1961).
59 SIMONS, D. J., DAY, E., GOODELL, H., and WOLFF, H. G. Experimental studies on headache: muscles of the scalp and neck as sources of pain. *Assoc. Res. nerv. Dis. Proc.*, **23**, 228–44 (1943).
60 SIMONS, D. J. and WOLFF, H. G. Studies on headache: mechanisms of chronic post-traumatic headache. *Psychsom. Med.*, **8**, 227 (1946).
61 SJAASTAD, O. and SJAASTAD, Ø. V. The histaminuria in vascular headache. *Acta Neurol. Scand.*, **46**, 331–42 (1970).
62 SOMERVILLE, B. W. The role of estradiol withdrawal in the etiology of menstrual migraine. *Neurology*, **22**, 355–65 (1972).
63 STEINHILBER, R. M., PEARSON, J. S., and RUSHTON, J. G. Some psychological considerations of histaminic cephalgia. *Proc. Staff Meet. Mayo Clin.*, **35**, 691–9 (1960).
64 THOMAS, J. E., ROOKE, E. D., and KVALE, W. F. The neurologist's experience with pheochromocytoma: a review of 100 cases. *J. Amer. med. Assoc.*, **197**, 754 (1966).
65 THONNARD-NEUMANN, E. Heparin in migraine headache. *Headache*, **13**, 49–64 (1973).
66 VANE, J. R. Inhibition of prostaglandin synthesis as a mechanism of action of aspirin-like drugs. *Nature* (*New Biol.*), **231**, 232 (1971).
67 VIJAYAN, N. and WATSON, C. Pericarotid syndrome. *Headache*, **18**, 244–254 (1978).
68 WALKER, A. E. Chronic post-traumatic headache. *Headache*, **5**, 67–72 (1965).
69 —— and JABLON, S. A followup of head-injured men of World War II. *J. Neurosurg*, **16**, 600 (1959).
70 WATERS, W. E. and O'CONNOR, P. J. Prevalence of migraine. *J. Neurol. Neurosurg. Psychiat.*, **30**, 613–16 (1975).
71 WELCH, K. M. A., CHABI, E., NELL, J. H., BARTOSH, K., CHEE, A. N. C., MATHEW, N. T., and ACHAR, V. S. Biochemical comparison of migraine and stroke. *Headache*, **16**, 160–7 (1976).

72 WHITTY, C. W. M. Familial hemiplegic migraine. *J. Neurol. Neurosurg. Psychiat.*, **16**, 172–7 (1953).
73 ——, HOCKADAY, J. M., and WHITTY, M. M. The effect of oral contraceptives on migraine. *Lancet*, **1**, 856–9 (1966).
74 WOLFF, H. G. and LENNOX, W. G. Cerebral circulation: 12. The effect on pial vessels of variations in the oxygen and carbon dioxide content of the blood. *Arch. Neurol.*, **23**, 1097 (1930).
75 ZIEGLER, D. K., HASSANEIN, R. S., HARRIS, D. and STEWART, R. Headache in a non-clinic twin population. *Headache*, **13**, 213–18 (1975).
76 ZUNG, W. W. K. A self-rating depression scale. *Arch. gen. Psychiat.*, **12**, 63–70 (1965).

7 Pathophysiology

Vascular changes

Neither the aetiology nor the pathogenesis of cluster headache is known. Why this condition affects males predominantly, exhibits unilateral symptoms, and occurs cyclically, remains unknown. Indeed, these examples hold the key to the aetiology of cluster headache. In recent years considerable progress has been made towards this goal. This chapter summarizes these findings.

Extracranial vasodilation

Horton[28] suspected that histamine-mediated extracranial vasodilatation was responsible for the symptoms of cluster headache. He based this on clinical features of the cluster attack:

1. Temporal artery swelling, engorgement of ocular soft tissue, conjunctival injection, nasal stuffiness, profuse watering of the eye and nose, and flushing. Indeed, the subcutaneous injection of 0·3–0·5 mg of histamine, a potent vasodilator, reproduced all signs and symptoms in such patients.
2. Alcohol, another vasodilating agent, was frequently reported to induce attacks.
3. Many patients reported that digital pressure over the ipsilateral temporal or common carotid artery reduced the pain, although temporarily.
4. Surface temperatures on the ipsilateral side of the head was 1–3°C warmer than that on the opposite side.
5. Vasoconstrictive agents were found to successfully abort or prevent cluster attacks.[12, 13, 17, 21, 61]

In fact, a selective action of ergotamine favouring the external carotid artery, was demonstrated by Saxena[54] and Spira, Mylecharne, and Lance[59] which lends support to Horton's conclusions regarding external carotid artery involvement in cluster headache.

Indirect evidence of extracranial dilatation during cluster attacks were demonstrated by Lance and Anthony[38] where facial thermography revealed increased ipsilateral heat in three of five patients, during attacks.

Kunkle, Pfeiffer, Wilhoit, and Hamrick[37] concluded that dilatation of external carotid artery branches was the principal contributor to the pain of cluster headache. During cluster attacks, two patients were subjected to controlled increases of intracranial pressure by the intrathecal injection of normal saline. Kunkle had earlier noted that this procedure eased the headaches of intracranial vasodilatation.[10] But in neither case was cluster pain relieved by this procedure. He also found that the head-jolt movement accentuated pain in several other patients, suggesting the possibility of internal carotid artery involvement, Ekbom[14] reported that rotary head-jolt had no effect on pain in 58·6 per cent of patients, improved it in 24 per cent, and caused exacerbation in 17·2 per cent. He also found that the *Valsalvor* manoeuvre had little effect on most of 22 patients subjected to this procedure. These findings indicated that involvement of intracranial arteries was unlikely. He also found that an equal number of patients experienced improvement or worsening of pain, following ipsilateral superficial temporal artery compression, but the majority of patients improved after digital compression of the carotid artery. Hence, it would appear that although the external carotid artery is involved in cluster pain, an internal carotid artery component is also present.

Internal carotid artery constriction

Hørven, Nornes, and Sjaastad[29] recorded increased pulse-synchronous indentation pulse waves on the symptomatic side during cluster headache attacks, in several patients. This result suggests involvement of the internal carotid artery system in cluster pain.

Broch, Hørven, Nornes, Sjaastad, and Tønsuma[6] demonstrated increased ipsilateral pulse-synchronous changes in eye tension using dynamic tonometry in three cases during cluster attacks. In one case, however, where they obtained simultaneous electromagnetic flowmetry from both internal carotid arteries, no change in blood-flow between sides was observed. It should be noted that placement of flowmeter probes were quite proximal (1 cm cranial to the carotid sinus) and could conceivably have been insensitive to more distal carotid artery changes.

Sjaastad, Rootwelt, and Hørven[56] measured cutaneous blood-flow by an isotope wash-out method on symptomatic and contralateral sides of the forehead in six patients during attack and interval phases of cluster periods. Although lowest cutaneous blood-flow values were found on the ipsilateral side during attacks, the differences were not significant. Conversely, dynamic tonometry revealed increased pulse synchronous amplitudes on the symptomatic side during attacks. They concluded that, although this evidence did not allow for deductions regarding total blood-flow through the eye, vasoconstriction occurring in more distal segments of the intraocular vessels could induce proximal vasodilatation as an effort to overcome increased resistance to the blood-flow.

Ekbom and Greitz[15] sought to compare differences of carotid artery size, in relation to bony structures of the skull, between cluster and non-cluster individuals. Eighteen patients (13 men and 5 women), 25–62 years of age, were investigated by angiography, performed by precutaneous puncture of either the internal or common carotid artery. Diameter measurements of the internal carotid artery were obtained at extradural and intradural cross-sections, and at levels through the carotid canal, close to its external aperture. Measurements of the middle cerebral arteries were also included. Similar measurements were made of 122 control patients for comparison.

They found that of 18 cluster patients, 4 males had generalized ectasia of all cerebral arteries. In addition, two women had questionable ectatic changes. Two of four males with ectasia were further examined by vertebral or aortocervical angiography; both exhibited ectatic cerebral vessels. Curiously, a female patient who 19 years previously, had a negative aortocervical angiogram, now showed evidence of these ectatic changes. She had been in remission for 17 years.

The mean values of various measurements of cerebral arteries were all greater in the cluster group when compared to controls. However, after correction for sex and skull size, no significant differences were noted for all but two measurements; the middle meningeal artery and the internal carotid artery at the level of the carotid canal near its external aperture.

Their findings were of great importance in one patient who had experienced a cluster attack soon after the initial carotid angiography had been performed. Second and third angiograms were obtained a few minutes after the attack onset, and just prior to the termination of attack, respectively. Soon after the attack onset, localized narrowing of the extradural part of the internal carotid artery was observed, distal to its exit from the carotid canal; and the ophthalmic artery was markedly dilated. On the third examination, narrowing had spread proximally to the lower part of the carotid canal (Plate 1).

They concluded that arterial narrowing was due either to spasm or oedema of the vessel wall, favouring the former explanation because of its rapid onset. They commented, however, that spastic contraction of the artery in the bony canal would have caused a vacuum effect between artery and bone, and ordinarily can be visualized radiographically. They pointed out that in two cases described by Walsh and O'Doherty,[62] where angiography was performed during ophthalmoplegic attacks, narrowing of the internal carotid artery in the cavernous sinus was found, and interpreted as an oedematous phenomenon. Similar findings had been reported by Bickerstaff[5] and appear to confirm the contention of Kunkle and Anderson[36] and Nieman and Hurwitz[46] that the minor eye signs of cluster attacks result from oculosympathetic paresis. Thus, during cluster attack, a segment of the internal carotid artery within the carotid canal constructs, becomes oedematous, expands, and compresses the accompanying sympathetic plexus to cause an oculo-sympathetic paresis or partial Horner's syndrome. Interestingly, in one patient who had been operated on because of intractable pain, Horton[27] found an enlarged, torturous middle cerebral artery. Nieman and Hurwitz[46] reported no abnormalities on angiography in six patients with cluster headache.

Considering the possibility of internal-carotid artery involvement in cluster, we studied supraorbital and frontal artery blood flow changes in cluster headache patients.[34] Blood-flow velocity in these arteries reflect internal carotid artery patency and are readily studied by the non-invasive Doppler flow examination.[7] Facial thermography was also incorporated as an adjunct to the Doppler flow examination.

The Doppler instrument used was the Parks Directional Doppler model 806–C. With the patient in the recumbent position, recordings from a Burdick EK-3 machine, were obtained from probe sites over the supraorbital and frontal arteries on each side before and after temporal artery compression. Although absolute flow velocity was not calculated, relative values were obtained by measuring the distance between the zero line and the bottom (diastolic foot) of the pulse wave, and expressed in millimetres. The mean flow velocity of frontal and supraorbital arteries were obtained on each side and compared. Each patient served as his own control. Facial thermography was performed in a temperature-regulated room using an

AGA Thermal Vision 750 colour camera. Patients were photo-graphed before and after temporal artery compression on each side. Thermography was performed between 30 minutes and one hour following Doppler examination.

In an attempt to ascertain the credibility of visualizing arterial heat by thermographic examination, a thermographic photograph was ob-tained of the radial artery region in one subject. As seen in Plate 2(a), radial artery heat was indeed delineated, and disappeared following tourniquet occlusion of radial artery blood-flow (Plate 2(b)).

This study was performed in three parts:

1. Doppler flow examination of 15 patients during their cluster periods, but headache-free;
2. Doppler flow examination in five patients during cluster attacks;
3. Doppler and thermographic examination in 20 patients during the cluster period, but headache-free.

In no case was thermography performed during an attack.

Thermographic examination was performed in a manner similar to that of the Doppler flow examination, that is, before and after right, then left, temporal artery compression. The frontal and supraorbital arteries are terminal branches of the ophthalmic artery, which in turn, is a branch of the internal carotid artery. The supraorbital artery anastomoses with the superficial temporal artery above the eye. Compression of the temporal artery therefore, results in an augmentation of supraorbital artery flow, as a reflection of the increased flow through the internal carotid artery.

Results of the first part of the study revealed that of 15 patients with right-sided headache, the supraorbital and frontal mean flow velocities were higher on the left, in 9 (60 per cent). Of 11 patients with left-sided headache, higher values were obtained on the right side in 9 (81·8 per cent), as seen in Table 7.1. In all, 18 of 26

Table 7.1 Frequency of higher Doppler flow values in relation to side of headaches in 26 cluster patients during active but non-headache state

Headache side	Side of higher mean flow velocity		
	R N (per cent)	L N (per cent)	Equal N (per cent)
Right	4 (26·7)	9 (60·0)	2 (13·3)
Left	9 (81·8)	2 (18·2)	0

(69·2 per cent) had higher flow values on the contralateral side ($p < 0.05$), as shown in Table 7.2.

Table 7.2   Mean Doppler flow values (mm) in relation to headache and non-headache side

	Contralat. > ipsilat.	Ipsilat. > contralat.	Sides equal
Side	$N = 18$ (69·2 per cent)	$N = 6$ (23·1 per cent)	$N = 2$ (7·7 per cent)
Contralateral	17·92	15·63	13·3
Ipsilateral	12·22	19·46	13·3
Difference	5·70	3·83	0·00

In the second part, five patients were examined during the early phase of the attack at 10–15 minutes, 20–30 minutes, and 45–60 minutes following ergotamine (sublingual) administration. Three had right-sided, and two, left-sided attacks. The difference in mean flow velocity between sides was plotted in relation to the stage of attack and side of cluster. Greater flow values were found on the contralateral side in both right and left-sided cluster patients, at the onset of attack. Ten to 15 minutes following ergotamine

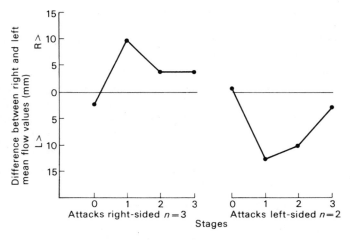

FIG. 7.1   Flow value difference between sides plotted against attack and post-ergotamine stages; where Stage 0 represents attack onset; Stages 1–3 represents 10–15, 20–30, and 45–60 minutes, post-ergotamine administration, respectively. [From Kudrow.[34]]

administration, a marked ipsilateral flow increase was noted in both right and left-sided cluster groups, increasing the difference between sides; flow from the contralateral side changed little. Thirty minutes after ergotamine administration, flow contracted somewhat on both sides with greater reduction ipsilaterally, narrowing the difference between sides. Forty-five to 60 minutes post-ergotamine, right and left flow values continued to narrow in both groups, approaching the zero line (Fig. 7.1).

In part 3 of our study, 20 asymptomatic patients in active cluster periods were evaluated by Doppler flow and thermographic examinations. These patients were classified in three groups:

1. Untreated (7 patients);
2. Unsuccessfully treated (6 patients);
3. Successfully treated (7 patients).

In Group 1, agreement between Doppler and thermographic results was 71 per cent, showing a higher contralateral flow (Table 7.3). Typical thermal changes, before and after temporal artery

Table 7.3   Doppler and thermographic differences between sides in untreated cluster patients during an interim period

Patient no.	Age	Sex	Cluster type and side	Doppler flow difference (mm)	Temperature difference (C)
1	36	M	episodic L	R > L 2·5	R > L 2·75
2	26	M	episodic R	R > L 10·0†	L > R 0·50
3	23	M	chronic L	R > L 22·5	R > L 0·50
4	54	M	episodic R	L > R 17·5	L > R 3·75
5	21	F	episodic R	L > R 7·5	Equal†
6	46	M	episodic R	L > R 20·0	L > R 1·50
7	35	M	episodic L	R > L 2·5	R > L 0·50

† Ipsilateral side equal to or greater than contralateral side.

compression, in a left-sided cluster patient, is demonstrated in Plate 3. In the pre-compression thermogram, left supraorbital heat is diminished, and increases, following left temporal artery compression. There also appears to be some shunting from left to right, across anastomosing frontal arteries. Less dramatic changes are seen following compression of the contralateral (right) temporal artery. Augmentation is evidenced by an increase in heat along the supraorbital distribution, but these changes are not as dramatic as that seen on the ipsilateral side following left temporal artery compression (Plate 3).

In the second group (unsuccessfully treated), 4 of 4 patients showed higher Doppler flow velocities on the contralateral side. Of 6 patients studied thermographically, 5 of 6 (83 per cent) and higher thermal values, contralaterally (Table 7.4).

Table 7.4   Doppler and thermographic differences between sides in unsuccessfully treated cluster patients during an interim period

Patient no.	Age	Sex	Cluster type and side	Medication used	Doppler flow difference (mm)	Temperature difference (C)
8	71	M	Episodic R	Ergotamine	L > R 20·0	L > R 0·50
9	44	M	Episodic L	Epinephrine	R > L 17·5	L > R 0·50†
10	30	M	Episodic R	Sansert	L > R 20·0	L > R 0·50
11	63	M	Episodic L	Ergotamine	R > L 7·5	R > L 1·50
12	36	M	Episodic R	Ergotamine‡	Not tested	L > R 0·50
13	30	M	Episodic L	Prednisone	Not tested	R > L 0·50

† Ipsilateral side equal to or greater than contralateral side.
‡ PRN medication–all others, prophylactic use.

Conversely, all 7 patients in Group 3 (successfully treated) revealed greater supraorbital heat on the ipsilateral side. Doppler examination revealed similar results, although less dramatically; 4 of 6 (67 per cent), had higher flow velocity values on the ipsilateral side (Table 7.5).

Table 7.5   Doppler and thermographic differences between sides in successfully treated cluster patients during an interim period

Patient no.	Age	Sex	Cluster type and side	Medication used	Doppler flow difference (mm)	Temperature difference (C)
14	54	M	chronic L	Ergotamine	L > R 12·5†	L > R 3·50†
15	38	F	episodic L	Ergotamine	L > R 17·5†	L > R 1·50†
16	63	M	chronic L	Lithium	R > L 10·0	L > R 4·50†
17	66	F	chronic R	Ergotamine	L > R 12·5	R > L 1·50†
18	33	M	episodic L	Ergotamine‡	L > R 2·5†	L > R 4·00†
19	34	M	episodic L	Ergotamine§	L > R 7·5†	L > R 0·50†
20	36	M	episodic L	Lithium ergotamine‡	Not tested	L > R 2·50†

† Ipsilateral side equal to or greater than contralateral side.
‡ PRN medication–others used prophylactically.
§ Doppler and thermograph obtained one hour post-ergotamine.

From the foregoing results, untreated and unsuccessfully treated patients are expected to yield ipsilateral Doppler and thermographic findings opposite to those of successfully treated patients. This expectation was tested and found to be significant (Table 7.6).

Table 7.6 Frequency of expected ipsilateral Doppler and thermographic values for all groups

Medication response	Expected ipsilateral findings†	
	Doppler N	Thermography N
Untreated and unsuccessfully treated	10/11‡	11/13‡
Successfully treated	4/6	7/7‡
Total	14/17‡	18/20§

† Decreased flow velocity and arterial heat on headache side in untreated and unsuccessfully treated patients. Reversed, in successfully treated.
‡ $p = > 0.01$.   § $p = > 0.001$.

Regarding earlier thermographic findings in cluster headache, Friedman and Wood[18] reported that two-thirds of 112 patients with cluster headache had areas of dense coolness (cold spots) over ipsilateral supraorbital regions. Lance and Anthony[38] having observed this thermographic pattern in two patients during a cluster attack, described the changes as not unlike those found in patients with internal carotid artery stenosis or occlusion.

We were able to demonstrate a discrete cold spot, ipsilaterally in a right-sided cluster patient, following compression of the contralateral (left) temporal artery. As seen in Plate 4(a), the thermogram reveals an hourglass-shaped area of coolness on the ipsilateral (right) side. The supraorbital flow on this side is apparently diminished when compared to the contralateral side. Following left temporal artery compression (Plate 4(b)), left supraorbital heat increased, and through frontal artery anastomosis supplied right supraorbital vessels. The latter change narrowed the area of coolness on the right to create the isolated 'cold spot'.

The results of our study indicate that ipsilateral ophthalmic-supraorbital arterial flow may be diminished during interim and attack states of cluster headache. It corroborates the finding of segmental constriction or spasm in the internal carotid artery region, as demonstrated by Ekbom and Greitz.[15]

During the cluster attack, temporal artery dilatation may be a passive and painless response to decrease ophthalmic artery flow, and not the cause of cluster pain. Indeed, the non-throbbing cluster pain is clearly distinct and different from the pulsatile temporal pain of migraine. Recently, Sakai and Meyer[53] compared temporal artery flow values between headache-free and attack states in seven patients with cluster headache. Although they demonstrated an almost five-fold increase in ipsilateral extracranial blood-flow during the attack, contralateral flow also increased by almost four times. Hence, if temporal artery dilatation is solely responsible for cluster pain, one would expect a bilateral pain distribution. Furthermore, in patients with atheromatous occlusion or partial occlusion of an internal carotid artery, ipsilateral temporal artery enlargement commonly occurs and it is painless.[16]

In the second part of our study we demonstrated that during a cluster attack, 10 minutes following ergotamine administration, ipsilateral supraorbital arterial flow velocity increased coincident to pain reduction.[34] To help explain this finding, the action of ergotamine on blood vessels is reviewed.

Aellig[1] studied the action of ergotamine on the circulatory system in 1967. He and Berde[2] also reported on the effects of other natural and synthetic ergot compounds on the peripheral vascular bed. In the latter study the limbs of dogs were perfused *in situ* with blood taken from the abdominal aorta and fed into the femoral arteries. Vascular resistance was determined on the basis of recorded changes in perfusion pressure. Changes in vascular resistance following infusion of ergot alkaloids in the untreated (control) limbs represented the peripheral vascular effects of these alkaloids. Alpha adrenergic blocking effects of the ergot alkaloids were determined by short infusions of noradrenalin in each femoral artery, before and after infusion of the ergot alkaloids. They found that all the alkaloids were similar, in that vasoconstriction was elicited when the resistance of the vessels were low, and vasodilatation occurred when vascular resistance was high. They also found that the increased vascular resistance induced by norepinephrine was inhibited by all alkaloids.[2]

These results provide an explanation why ergotamine had caused an increase in the ipsilateral supraorbital flow during cluster headache. It would appear that in an active cluster state, the vascular resistance on the side of cluster is increased; as demonstrated in part l of this study. Hence administration of ergotamine would decrease vascular resistance and increase blood-flow.

Cerebral blood-flow changes

In one patient having a cluster attack, Norris, Hachinski, and Cooper[47] demonstrated an increased ipsilateral CBF, ten minutes after ergotamine administration. Since ergotamine does not affect the cerebral vessels directly, their finding suggests that increased CBF occurred as a result of increased internal carotid artery flow. It also suggests an auto-regulatory impairment.

Of special interest in this regard, were the findings of Sakai and Meyer.[53] They obtained CBF measurements from both hemispheres in five patients during attack and headache-free states. They found that during the attack period mean CBF of the contralateral hemisphere increased by 30 per cent, but only 13 per cent, ipsilaterally. Although it has been suggested that the increased CBF represents reactive hyperaemia,[47, 53] it is less clear why the high flow values are not equal, bilaterally. Could it be related to carotid flow asymmetry? Jennett, Miller, and Harper[30] reported that following unilateral carotid ligation, there is diminished reserve in the circulation of the ipsilateral hemisphere, resulting in a reduced auto-regulatory response to hypotension, hypoxia, and hypercapnia. This observation may explain the recent findings of Sakai and Meyer.[52] They found that during the cluster attack, cerebrovascular responses to carbon dioxide was impaired, and to oxygen, excessive.

Biochemical aspects

Histamine

Horton[25] suggested that cluster headache was associated with an unusual histamine sensitivity. This was based on clinical features and observation that subcutaneous administration of histamine 0·35 mg induced attacks identical to spontaneous attacks. Furthermore, he reported, that following an extended period of histamine desensitization, attacks tended to subside.[25] However, Dalessio[11] commented that attacks could be reproduced not only by histamine, but also by ingestion of alcohol, suggesting that these events may simply indicate an increased susceptibility of cranial arteries to diverse vasodilating agents, in these patients. He further cautions that, as with all periodic disorders, evaluation of prophylactic drugs may be difficult, in view of the occurrence of spontaneous remissions. Finally, he notes that improvement in headache after an elaborate programme of histamine desensitization has, by controlled experiments, not been shown to be due to a desensitizing effect of this agent.[11] (Unfortunately, he did not provide us with a reference.)

In a study of free histamine excretion, Sjaastad[55] found an increased urinary output in 3 of 6 patients during cluster attacks. Subsequently, Sjaastad and Sjaastad[57] determined urinary excretion of labelled histamine and its metabolites in migraine and cluster patients, following oral and subcutaneous administration of radioactive histamine. With the exception of one patient diagnosed as having CPH, results in all patients were normal.

Anthony and Lance[3] obtained blood histamine levels from 20 cluster patients during 22 attacks. Of these, 11 were induced by sublingual administration of nitroglycerine (1 mg), 5 by alcohol induction, and, in 6, headaches occurred spontaneously. One to four histamine blood samples were obtained from each patient during pre-headache, headache, and post-headache states. Histamine levels were found to be higher during headache than pre-headache periods in 19 of 22 attacks. The mean increase was 20·5 per cent; this difference was highly significant. They concluded that some of the clinical features associated with the cluster attack may be explained by the sudden rise of blood histamine.

Blood histamine changes were also evaluated in ten migraine patients. Histamine levels rose slightly during the headache period. Post-headache values were significantly higher than pre-headache values.[3]

Subsequently, Anthony et al.[4] reported their results on controlled trials of cimetidine (H_2 histamine receptor antagonist) alone, and in combination with an histamine H_1 receptor antagonist, chlorpheniramine, for prophylactic efficacy in cluster headache. They found that H_2-receptor blockade with cimetidine, even when combined with H_1-receptor blockers, was not superior to placebo. These negative results were interpreted as evidence, more against H_2-receptor involvement in cluster headache, than against histamine activation, since induced intracellular histamine does not act through receptors and remains inaccessible to histamine receptor blockade.

Hence, they concluded that the role of histamine in cluster headache is in no way refuted by the negative results of their study.[4]

Similar negative results were obtained in a more recent multicentre study (unpublished). Diamond, Graham, and Kudrow had evaluated a total of 60 cluster patients for response to histamine H_1 plus H_2 antagonists over a two-week trial period. All patients were in active cluster periods. Placebos were administered during the first and last four days. No significant responses were reported for either placebo or treatment periods.

Serotonin

Anthony and Lance[3] measured plasma serotonin levels in 20 cluster patients during 30 headaches; 13 attacks had occurred spontaneously, 12 were induced by sublingual nitroglycerin, and 5 induced by alcohol ingestion. No statistically significant differences were found for serotonin levels between the three periods. Among migraine patients, however, serotonin levels were significantly lower during the headache phase, than during pre-headache periods.

Autonomic nervous system

In 1959, Kunkle[35] proposed that cluster headache attacks result from parasympathetic storms involving the seventh and tenth cranial nerves; as evidenced by symptoms such as lacrimation, conjunctival injection, nasal congestion, and, in some cases, bradycardia. He obtained spinal fluid specimens from 14 patients during their cluster headache attacks, and in 7 patients with migraine. He found acetylcholine-like substances in the cerebral spinal fluid of four cluster patients. This substance was not found in the spinal fluid of any of the migraine patients.

Gardner, Stowell, and Dutlinger[19] were also of the opinion that cluster headache resulted from parasympathetic activation specifically mediated through the greater superficial petrosal nerve. Actually, typical cluster attacks were induced upon stimulation of this nerve. Section of the greater superficial petrosal nerve in thirteen patients resulted in, failure in 25 per cent, partial success in 50 per cent, and an excellent outcome in 25 per cent.

Stowell[60] suggested that cluster headache is produced by efferent impulses from the superficial petrosal nerves, arising in the parasympathetic nuclei of the hypothalamus. These nuclei are influenced by abnormal impulses arising from cortical and thalamic areas. When cortical control is inhibited during relaxation, efferent impulses passed down to the hypothalamus and then to the dorsal longitudinal fasciculus to the nuclei of the V, VII, and IX cranial nerves, and to the superior cervical sympathetic ganglion. He added that the chief flow passes over the VII cranial nerve. Impulses over the petrosal nerve produce vasodilatation of ophthalmic artery branches and adjacent arteries; and also flows to the sphenopalatine ganglion. Stowell[60] further reported that section of the greater superficial petrosal nerves in 32 cluster patients resistant to drug therapy, resulted in failure in only 12·5 per cent of patients. Of 28 patients who had obtained relief, recurrence was found in 53·6 per cent: 28·6 per cent after one year; 10·7 per cent after two years; and 14·3 per cent after three years follow-up. Resection of the first division of the V cranial nerve resulted in 'permanent' relief in 5 of 5 patients. He also observed that injection of the cervical sympathetic chain during cluster attacks, produced complete relief in four patients. Avulsion or alcohol block of the supraorbital nerves relieved attacks in 11 of 16 patients.[60]

In an attempt to interrupt the proximal parasympathetic outflow to the petrosal nerves, Sachs[51] sectioned the nervus intermedius in one patient who had had repeated petrosal nerve sections because of recurrent cluster headaches. The patient remained free of clusters during a ten-year follow-up period following section of the nervus intermedius, but suffered permanent unilateral nerve deafness and a loss of the sense of smell.

Bruyn, Bootsma, and Klawans[8] consider the primary abnormality in cluster headache as one involving the autonomic centres in the lower brain-stem. They considered the parasympathetic model too limited and untenable to explain cluster headache, in view of the finding of bradycardia during cluster attacks in some patients, and in one case, an associated systolic and diastolic hypertension. Thus, they hypothesized that cluster headache attacks are associated with central α-adrenergic paroxysms (both excitatory and inhibitory).

Electroencephalography, pneumoencephalography, and CAT scans

Stowell[60] reported that electroencephalography in 100 cluster patients was essentially normal. However, pneumoencephalography revealed mild to moderate left ventricular dilatation in 46 per cent. This was not found to be the case as reported by Russell, Nakstad, and Sjaastad.[49] They examined 28 cluster patients by computerized axial tomography (CT scan). Half of these patients had previously undergone pneumoencephalographic procedures. Of 14 patients, pneumoencephalography revealed borderline values of ventricular width in two, and showed slight cortical atrophy in one. CT scans of these patients were interpreted as normal. Of the remaining patients, CT scans were assessed as normal in all but one, who was found to have slight central atrophy. None of the CT scans showed evidence of low density areas of the cerebral parenchyma.

Hormonal changes

Ekbom[12] and Olivarius[48] had reported an apparent relationship between cluster attacks and menstrual periods in one patient. However, in Ekbom's series[12] of 13 women with cluster headache, only one reported such a relationship. He also stated that although the majority of his patients had experienced remissions during pregnancy, one patient had observed the occurrence of cluster headache during two successive pregnancies.

Among our women with cluster headache, there appears to be no relationship, either between menstrual periods and attacks, or between pregnancy and remission. In migraine, on the other hand, there is little doubt that such an association exists.[58] Also, the influence of extrinsic oestrogens on migraine frequency has been established;[33] indeed, in response to altered oestrogen levels, significant histological changes in the uterine vasculature of migrainous women has been demonstrated.[22]

Is then, the influence of testosterone in cluster headache, a predominantly male disorder, similar to that of oestrogen in migraine, a predominantly female disorder? This question is important in that, both hormones affect vasomotor stability.[40] In addition, Graham[20] noted that cluster males appear to have exaggerated masculine characteristics.

For these reasons we measured plasma testosterone levels in 19 male patients, during active cluster and remission periods.[32] Patients were divided into two groups. In Group 1, three were in active periods and six in remission. In Group 2, six were in active periods and four were in remission. Blood samples from Group 1 patients were separated from those in Group 2, and plasma testosterone was determined in separate laboratories, respectively.

The mean testosterone value for active cluster males in Group 1 was found to be significantly lower than in the mean level for those in remission, ($t(7) = -1.896$; $p < 0.05$), or for normal controls, ($t(7) = -2.9627$; $p < 0.05$). Testosterone values of remission males were also significantly lower than normal controls ($t(5) = -3.9512$; $p < 0.01$) (Table 7.7). In Group 2, the mean testosterone value for

Table 7.7　Mean plasma testosterone levels from cluster and control males in group 1†

Subjects	N	Mean age	Testosterone levels mean $\pm$ SD (mg/100 ml)
Cluster patients			
Active period	3	43	238 ± 144
Remission period	6	51	$401 \pm 79\ddagger$
Controls	10	40	$530 \pm 181\S$

†Determination by Damon Laboratory.
‡ Active *VRS* remission—$t(7) = -1.896$; $p < 0.05$.
§ Active *VRS* controls—$t(2) = -2.9627$; $p < 0.05$.

active cluster males was significantly lower than mean values for cluster males in remission, ($t(8) = -3.7742$; $p < 0.005$), and normal controls ($t(5) = -23.7061$; ($p < 0.0005$). The mean testosterone level for cluster males in remission was lower than the control value, although this difference did not reach statistical significance (Table 7.8).

Table 7.8　Mean plasma testosterone levels from cluster and control males in group 2†

Subjects	N	Mean age	Testosterone level mean $\pm$ SD (mg/100 ml)
Cluster patients			
Active period	6	41	425 ± 38
Remission period	4	44	$675 \pm 160\ddagger$
Controls	33	42	$796 \pm 277\S$

†Determination by Nichols Institute.
‡ Active remission—$t(8) = -3.7742$; $p < 0.005$.
§ Active controls—$t(5) = -23.7061$; $p < 0.0005$.

These preliminary results show that testosterone levels are lower during the active cluster period, when compared to the remission period; but not low enough to induce changes in secondary male characteristics or libido. Low testosterone levels, however, are associated with psychic symptoms, including depression, tearfulness, lassitude, fatigue, and inability to concentrate.[63] These symptoms in addition to vasomotor changes are generally observed among cluster patients during active cluster periods. Similar symptoms have been reported by Heller and Myers[24] during the male climacteric, when associated with elevated urine gonadotrophins; improvement in symptomatology was obtained following administration of testosterone.[24]

More recently, Nelson[45] compared plasma testosterone levels between 30 cluster and 30 classical migraine males, and found no difference between these two groups. However, testosterone values were abnormally low in 22 per cent of cluster patients. Approximately the same frequency of abnormally low values were found in the classical migraine group.[45] Unfortunately, a comparison was not made between cluster patients in active and in remission periods. In only two cases, blood samples had been obtained during active and remission periods. In three other cases, samples were obtained during remission but not active periods. (Table 7.9)

Elevated testosterone values were found in two of four women sampled. The remaining two patients had values near upper limits of normal[45]. This finding may add credence to Graham's observation[20] that women with cluster tend to be somewhat more masculine. In spite of elevated testosterone levels, however, four women patients had neither masculine characteristics nor endocrine disturbances.

Nelson[45] speculated that the finding of lower testosterone levels in some cluster and migraine patients may be influenced by: the stage of cluster period in which samples are drawn, since patients tend to become debilitated and often lose weight during extensive periods of recurrent pain; excessive drug use; chronic illness states; or disturbed sleep patterns, since peak testosterone secretion often occurs in conjunction with REM sleep.

Lower testosterone levels during the active cluster period in some patients, suggest periodic dysfunction in the hypothalamic–pituitary–gonadal system. If LH levels were increased during this period, it would suggest gonadal dysfunction; decreased LH levels would be

Table 7.9   Plasma testosterone values in cluster and non-cluster headache males

Cluster headache					Non-cluster headache			
Case	Age	During headache	Headache-free	At end of cluster	Case	Age	During headache	Headache-free
1	72		552		1	39		177
2	21		441		2	51		606
3	50		763		3	43		591
4	27	531	556	550	4	42		231
5	25		331		5	55	568	699
6	66		543		6	28	331	
7	26		278		7	29		396
8	44		387	412	8	35	418	
9	38		414		9	62		320
10	50		542		10	52	451	
11	56		618		11	50		325
12	34		269		12	50		587
13	62		281		13	30		356
14	30		508		14	32		695
15	30		431		15	51		406
16	33		425		16	33		581
17	53		412		17	23		594
18	29		212		18	31		171
19	20	987	875		19	32		243
20	43		529		20	29		200
21	53	431	512		21	52	507	
22	32	375	360		22	27	787	638
23	46			480	23	23		566
24	39		610		24	26		644
25	47		234		25	29		468
26	53		555		26	30	277	334
27	38		361		27	21	581	431
28	43		424		28	23		281
29	57			655	29	47		162
30	23			481	30	31		518
Mean	41	631	460·4	515·6		36·7	490	431·5
Mean for all tests:			487·0					445·3

Normal range for testosterone: 300–850 ng/dl

From Nelson, R. F.[45] by courtesy of the author and editor.

suggestive of hypothalamic–pituitary dysfunction. In an attempt to determine the level at which dysfunction occurs, we obtained blood samples from five cluster patients during both active and remission periods, and measured testosterone, LH and testosterone binding globulin (TBG) levels. In addition, we tested for changes in prolactin, TSH, FSH, growth hormone, cortisol, T_3 and T_4 uptake, and reverse T_3. Specimens were obtained at the same time of the day from each patient during cluster and remission periods. All blood samples were collected, frozen, and determinations were made in the same run twice, by the Endocrine Science Laboratory.

In each case, testosterone and LH values were lower during cluster than remission periods. According to the binomial test, this difference

Table 7.10   Plasma testosterone, LH and TBG levels during active and remission periods of five cluster headache males

Patients†	Testosterone (mg/100 ml)		LH (MIU/ml)		TBG (µg/100 mg)	
	Active	Remiss.	Active	Remiss.	Active	Remiss.
1	451	514	6·9	8·0	0·8	0·8
2	298	478	7·1	19·0	0·9	1·0
3	395	455	12·7	18·3	1·0	1·2
4	595	929	11·7	—	1·2	1·3
5	656	793	10·0	16·0	1·3	1·0
Mean	479‡	633·8	9·68‡	15·33	1·04	1·06
	± 105·7	± 191·1	± 2·35	± 4·38	± 0·18	± 0·17

†Average age = 42.   ‡$p < 0.05$.

Table 7.11   Mean hormone levels of 5 cluster patients during active and remission periods

Hormones	Mean values‡	
	Active periods	Remission periods
Prolactin (ng/ml)	7·5 ± 3·69	6·3 ± 2·225
TSH (MIU/ml)	3·4 ± 0·89	3·9 ± 0·88
FSH (MIU/ml)	7·8 ± 2·09	8·3 ± 2·45
Growth hormone†		
Cortisol (µg/100 ml)	11·0 ± 3·55	11·5 ± 2·75
T_3 uptake	41·9	42·3
T_4 uptake	10·1	10·0
Reverse T_3	37·4	45·2

† < 1·0 ng/ml in 3/5, active; 4/5, remission.
‡No significant differences between periods.

was significant ($p < 0.05$). Mean values from active cluster was also significantly lower than that from the remission periods as determined by the t test ($p < 0.05$); while testosterone binding globulin was found to be unchanged (Table 7.10). Values for other hormones tested, as seen in Table 7.11, showed no significant difference between active cluster and remission periods.

The finding of decreased plasma testosterone and LH levels, occurring together, suggests impairment in the hypothalamic–pituitary axis, and specifically in the hypothalamus, since other anterior pituitary hormone levels remained unchanged.

Hypothesis of the pathogenesis of cluster headache

Most of the data presented in this chapter concerns, more, the events associated with the cluster attack than the cluster condition. An approach to the question of pathogenesis requires examination of issues concerning male predominance, and of the cyclic nature inherent to this disorder.

Male predominance

Studies on familial incidence in cluster headache populations suggest an absence of genetic susceptibility. Although male prevalence in itself may indicate sex-linked or sex-influenced genetic determination, as in colour blindness or haemophilia, the frequency of cluster among fathers and sons (greater than among mothers and sons) would rule it out.

If male hormones played the major role in male predominance, then cluster headache would be commonplace in the male population; and, of course, it is not. Thus, since neither genetic nor hormonal factors appear to be the major influence of male predominance, then other environmental factors, peculiar to males, should be considered.

The initial injury. The second issue that closely relates to pathogenesis is the cyclic nature of cluster headache. Cycles are observed at two levels; circannual cluster periods and circadian timing of attacks. It is hardly a coincidence that both cluster periods and attacks are cyclic in nature. It implies a dysfunction of central regulating mechanisms responsible for rhythmic activity. Specifically, if, as suspected, hypothalamic and limbic centres regulate rhythmic secretions of biogenic amines, which in effect, activate or inhibit autonomic and other nervous system pathways, then injury to these centres may result in asynchronous discharges and disrhythmic nervous function.†

The following hypothesis is limited by the sparsity of information regarding the pain mechanism in cluster headache, and control mechanisms of biogenic rhythms. It therefore requires a series of assumptions that are, as yet, unsupported by substantive data.

Initial injury to hypothalamic-limbic centres may result as a consequence of life-style factors peculiar to some young men. The male psyche, at an age between the teens and late-twenties, is one mixed with bravado and uncertainty, responsibility and self-indulgence, and, deliberation and impulsiveness. His problems and behaviour are qualitatively different from that of women. Hence, periods of excessive drinking, sleep deprivation, drug use, and other potentially damaging experiences, may cause toxic or metabolic injury to some brain centres at neuronal receptor levels. Perhaps concomitant insults arising from anaesthesia, high fever, medication use, or conditions causing hypoxaemia potentiates the injurious effects of other experiences.

Cluster periods (Fig. 7.2)

To explain circannual occurrence of cluster periods, this hypothesis requires three assumptions. It assumes *first*, that rhythm regulatory centres operate with diminished capacity; *second*, that when challenged, either by intrinsic or extrinsic stimuli, these centres fail to respond appropriately; and *third*, that such inadequate responses cause dyssynchronous secretion of peripheral hormones central biogenic amines, and other biochemicals, resulting in ineffective or inappropriate functions of the autonomic nervous system and other neuronal pathways.

Circannual rhythmicity of various physiologic functions has been established. Moreover, some annual rhythms occur solely in males. As an example, annual rhythms of EEG patterns in man, has been reported.[23] Seasonal rhythmicity[31,44] and shifting circadian rhythms[43] have also been demonstrated in male laboratory rats.

Returning to the above assumptions, the hypothesis holds that

---

† Since the time of writing, this concept has been also reported by Medina, J. L., Diamond, S., and Fareed, J. (*Headache* **19**, 309–22, 1979).

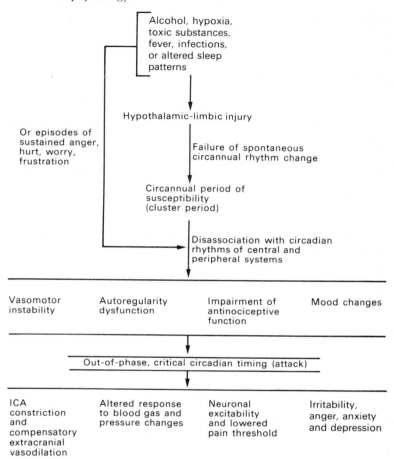

FIG. 7.2   Hypothetical schema of the pathogenesis of cluster headache.

as a result of injury to central rhythm regulating mechanisms, normal circannual rhythm shifts are abolished or modified. This heralds the onset of circannual cluster periods, in which dyssynchronous biological rhythms prevail. Such changes could result in vasomotor instability, auto-regulatory dysfunction, impairment of antinociceptive function, and mood changes, and would persist for the duration of the cluster period. Hence, cluster periods may occur spontaneously, or may require additional stimuli to provoke its onset.

Cluster period onset has been associated with alcohol use[39] and fever or infection.[26] We have found two other conditions that appear with considerable regularity in association with the cluster period onset. The first concerns sleep–wake cycle change, associated with prolonged periods of anger, 'hurt', worry, or frustration, and the second, exposure to toxic substances. Examples of both conditions are described in the following case reports.

Case 7.1. A 40-year-old male attorney began having cluster headaches at age 19, upon starting his university studies. Cluster periods, that lasted two to three months, recurred each year for the following eight years. They ceased to occur after his first year in private law practice, and he remained in remission for the next 13 years.

He had always considered himself a 'night person', suspecting that forced awakening early in the morning during his school years was responsible for the clusters. After his first year in private practice, he had scheduled his office hours during time periods which did not necessitate early arising; hence, he believed, enjoying a remission period for 13 years.

Confident that he was forever 'cured' of his headaches, he extended his office hours to an earlier time period since he wished to enjoy free afternoons, for recreation. In mid-April of 1978, he began to awaken one hour earlier each morning. And coincident to this change he gained an additional morning hour as the result of 'daylight savings time' change. In effect, he was awakening two hours earlier than usual.

Six weeks later, he experienced his first cluster period since the last episode 13 years ago. Despite changing his hours back to later times of awakening, the cluster period lasted four and one-half months, during which time he experienced attacks occurring twice a day with clockwork regularity, at approximately 9 a.m. and 9 p.m.

The patient was questioned in great detail regarding other changes that could have been associated with the new cluster onset. He admitted that for six weeks prior to the cluster onset he experienced a sustained rage and feeling of helplessness, arising from conflict with a building contractor who had fled with a sizeable down-payment for home remodelling construction.

Case 7.2. Two middle-aged male patients who were being followed at our clinic, met each other, coincidentally, in the clinic's waiting-room, after not having seen each other for more than 25 years. One patient had chronic cluster headache and the other, episodic. Both men had been employed in a machine-shop 25 years ago. They were involved in a curious incident; a fire had erupted in their work area, and both men extinguished the fire; and each had used carbon tetrachloride fire extinguishers (subsequently removed from the market because of pulmonary and hepatic toxicity). Six weeks following the incident, one man began to experience chronic cluster headaches and three months after the incident, the second man developed episodic cluster headaches.

Although coincidence can account for the above case report, it is possible that exposure to carbon tetrachloride may have been responsible for cluster headache in both patients.

Cyclic cluster attacks (Fig. 7.2)

The cluster period is a period of susceptibility in which optimal endocrine, neuronal, vasomotor, and emotional functions are compromised. Since circadian variations in peripheral organ systems are modified by circannual or seasonal rhythms,[41] then abnormal or inappropriate function of the latter would affect the integrity of the circadian rhythm, and ultimately induce dyssynchronous biochemical and neuronal discharge.

Circadian rhythms have been established for numerous physiological functions in humans.[42] A higher incidence of disorders has been reported by Rutenfranz,[50] among 'shift workers' who exhibit altered biological rhythms. Cahn, Folk, and Huston[9] stated that disassociation of circadian rhymicity in human beings may lead to loss of health.

It is proposed that the cyclic cluster attack conforms to circadian timing, and represents that time in which critical circadian function fails. 'Out-of-phase' secretory rhythms disrupt agonist–antagonist homeostasis of various systems, including vasomotor, cerebrovascular autoregulatory, antinociceptive, and emotional. Pathophysiologic changes resulting from this, have been detailed earlier in this chapter. They include internal and external carotid artery changes, cerebral vascular dysauto-regulation, and biochemical and hormonal alterations (Fig. 7.2).

References

1 AELLIG, W. H. Periphers kreislaufwiakungen von Ergotamin Dihydroergotamin und 1-Methyl-ergotamin an der innervieten, perfundierten Hinterextremität des Hundes. *Helv. Physiol. Acta*, **25**, 374–9 (1967).

2 —— and Berde, B. Studies of the effect of natural and synthetic polypeptide type ergot compounds on a peripheral vascular bed. *Brit. J. Pharmacol.*, **36**, 561–70 (1969).

3 ANTHONY, M. and LANCE, J. W. Histamine and serotonin in cluster headache. *Arch. Neurol.*, **25**, 225–31 (1971).

4 ——, LORD, G. D. A., and LANCE, J. W. Controlled trials of cimetidine in migraine and cluster headache. *Headache*, **18**, 261–4 (1978).

5 BICKERSTAFF, E. R. Ophthalmoplegic migraine. *Rev. Neurol.*, **110**, 582 (1964).

6 BROCH, A., HØRVEN, I., NORNES, H., SJAASTAD, O., and TØNSUMA, A. Studies of cerebral and ocular circulation in a patient with cluster headache. *Headache*, **10**, 1–13 (1970).

7 BROCKENBROUGH, E. C. *Screening for the prevention of strokes: use of a Doppler flowmeter*. Parks Electronics, Beaverton, Oregon (1970).

8 BRUYN, G. W., BOOTSMA, B. K., and KLAWANS, H. L. Cluster headache and bradycardia. *Headache*, **16**, 11–15 (1976).

9 CAHN, H. A., FOLK, G. E., and HUSTON, P. E. Age comparison of human day–night physiological differences. *Aerospace Med.* (June 1968).

10 DALESSIO, D. J. *Wolff's headache and other head pain*. (3rd edn.), pp. 157–171. Oxford University Press, New York (1972).

11 ——. *Wolff's headache and other head pain*. (3rd edn.), pp. 349–50. Oxford University Press, New York (1972).

12 EKBOM, K. A. Ergotamine tartrate orally in Horton's 'histaminic cephalgia' (also called Harris's 'ciliary neuralgia'). *Acta Psychiat. Scand. (Suppl.)*, **46**, 106–13 (1947).

13 EKBOM, K. Prophylactic treatment of cluster headache with a new serotonin antagonist, *BC* 105. *Acta Neurol. Scand.* **45**, 601–10 (1969).

14 ——. Some observations on pain in cluster headache. *Headache*, **13**, 219–25 (1975).

15 —— and GREITZ, T. Carotid angiography in cluster headache. *Acta Radiol. Diagnos.*, **10**, 177–86 (1970).

16 FISHER, C. M. Facial pulses in internal carotid artery occlusion. *Neurology*, **20**, 476–8 (1970).

17 FRIEDMAN, A. P. and ELKIND, A. H. Appraisal of methysergide in treatment of vascular headaches of migraine type. *J. Amer. med. Assoc.*, **184**, 125–30 (1963).

18 —— and WOOD, E. H. Thermography in vascular headache. In *Medical thermography* (ed. S. Uema), pp. 80–4. Brentwood Publishers, Los Angeles (1976).

19 GARDNER, W. J., STOWELL, A., and DUTLINGER, R. Resection of the greater superficial petrosal nerve in the treatment of unilateral headache. *J. Neurosurg.*, **4**, 105–14 (1947).

20 GRAHAM, J. R. Cluster headache. *Headache*, **11**, 175–85 (1972).

21 ——. Methysergide for prevention of headache: experience in five hundred patients over three years. *New Engl. J. Med.*, **270**, 67–72 (1964).

22 GRANT, E. C. G. Relation between headache from oral contraception and development of endometrial arterioles. *Brit. med. J.*, **3**, 402–5 (1968).

23 GUTJAHR, V. L., KÜNKEL, H., and MACHLEIDT, W. Jahresrhythmen der häufigkeit Elektroenzephalograyhischer merkmale. *Arzneim-Forsch Drug. Res.*, **28**(11), 1857–61 (1978).

24 HELLER, C. G. and MYERS, G. B. The male climacteric, its symptomatology, diagnosis and treatment. *J. Amer. med. Assoc.*, **126**, 472–7 (1944).

25 HORTON, B. T. Histaminic cephalgia: differential diagnosis and treatment. *Proc. Mayo Clin.*, **31**, 325 (1956).

26 ——. Histaminic cephalgia linked with respiratory infection. *Headache*, **4**, 228–36 (1964).

27 ——. The use of histamine in the treatment of specific types of headaches. *J. Amer. med. Assoc.*, **116**, 377 (1941).

28 ——, MacLEAN, A. R., and CRAIG, W. M. A New syndrome of vascular headache: results of treatment with histamine: preliminary report. *Proc. Mayo Clin.*, **14**, 257–60 (1939).

29 HØRVEN, I., NORNES, H., and SJAASTAD, O. Different corneal indentation pulse patterns in cluster headache and migraine. *Neurology*, **22**, 92–8 (1972).

30 JENNETT, B., MILLER, J. D., and HARPER, A. M. Experimental investigation of carotid ligation in primates (*Excerpta Medica*). In: *Effect of carotid artery surgery on cerebral blood flow—Clinical and experimental studies*, pp. 111–22. Elsevier/North-Holland Biomedical Press, Amsterdam, (1976).

31 KINSON, G. A. and LIU, C-C. Further evidence of inherent testicular rhythms in the laboratory rat. *J. Endocrinol.*, **56**, 337–8 (1973).

32 KUDROW, L. Plasma testosterone levels in cluster headache: preliminary results. *Headache*, **16**, 28–31 (1976).

33 ——. The relationship of headache frequency to hormonal use in migraine. *Headache*, **15**, 36–40 (1975).

34 ——. Thermographic and Doppler flow asymmetry in cluster headache. Presented at the 2nd International Migraine Symposium, London, Sept. 1978. *Headache* **19**, 204–8 (1979).

35 KUNKLE, E. C. Acetylcholine in the mechanism of headaches of the migraine type. *Arch. Neurol. Psychiat.* (*Chicago*), **84**, 135 (1959).

36 —— and ANDERSON, W. B. (1960). Dual mechanisms of eye signs of headache in cluster pattern. *Trans. Amer. Neurol. Assoc.*, **85**, 75 (1960).

37 ——, PFEIFFER, J. P. JR., WILHOIT, W. M., and HAMRICK, L. W. JR. Recurrent brief headache in 'cluster pattern'. *Trans. Amer. Neurol.*, **77**, 240–3 (1952).

38 LANCE, J. W. and ANTHONY, M. Thermographic studies in vascular headache. *Med. J. Aust.*, **1**, 240 (1971).

39 LOVSHIN, L. L. Clinical caprices of histaminic cephalgia. *Headache*, **1**, 3–6 (1961).

40 McCULLOGH, E. P. Climacteric—male and female. *Cleveland Clin. Quart.*, **13**, 166–76 (1946).

41 MAYERSBACH, VON HV. Die Zeitstrukture des organisms. *Arzneim–Forsch/Drug Res.*, **28**(11), 1809–72 (1978).

42 MILLS, J. N. Human circadian rhythms. *Physiol. Rev.*, **46**, 128–70 (1966).

43 MOCK, E. J. and FRANKEL, A. I. A shifting circannual rhythm in serum testosterone concentration in male laboratory rats. *Biol. reproduction*, **19**, 927–30 (1978).

44 ——, KAMEL, F., WRIGHT, W. W. and FRANKEL, A. I. Seasonal rhythm in plasma testosterone and luteinizing hormone of the male laboratory rat. *Nature*, **256**, 6!–3, (1975).

45 NELSON, R. F. Testosterone levels in cluster and non-cluster migrainous headache patients. *Headache*, **18**, 265–7 (1978).

46 NIEMAN, E. A. and HURWITZ, L. J. Ocular sympathetic palsy in periodic migrainous neuralgia. *J. Neurol. Neurosurg. psychiat.*, **24**, 369 (1961).

47 NORRIS, J. W., HACHINSKI, V. C., and COOPER, P. W. Cerebral blood flow changes in cluster headache. *Acta Neurol. Scand.*, **54**, 371–4 (1976).

48 OLIVARIUS, B. DE FINE. Periodik neuralgiform hemikrani, et karakteristisk vaskulaert hovedtine syndrom. *Maanedsskr. prakt. Laegeg. soc. Med.*, 155–65 (1966).

49 RUSSELL, D., NAKSTAD, P., and SJAASTAD, O. Cluster headache-pneumoencephalographic and cerebral computerized axial tomography findings. *Headache*, **18**, 272–3 (1978).

50 RUTENFRANZ VON J. Schichtarbeit und biologische rhythmik. *Arzneim–Forsch./Drug Res.*, **28**(11), 1867–72 (1978).

51 SACHS, E. JR. The role of the nervus intermedius in facial neuralgia. Report of four cases with observations on the pathways for taste, lacrimation, and pain in the face. *J. Neurosurg.*, **23**, 54–60 (1968).

52 SAKAI, F. and MEYER, J. S. Abnormal cerebrovascular reactivity in patients with migraine and cluster headache. Presented at Twenty-first Annual Meeting, American Association for the Study of Headache, Boston, June, 1979. *Headache* **19**, 257–66 (1979).

53 —— and ——. Regional cerebral hemodynamics during migraine and cluster headaches measured by the ^{133}Xe inhalation method. *Headache*, **18**, 122–32 (1978).

54 SAXENA, P. R. The effect of antimigraine drugs on the vascular responses of 5-hydroxytryptamine and related biogenic substances on the external carotid bed of dogs: possible pharmacological implications to their antimigraine action. *Headache*, **12**, 44–53 (1972).

55 SJAASTAD, O. Kinin-OG histaminiunders ø kelser ved migrene, in *Kliniske aspekter i migrene forshningen*, pp. 61–9. Norlundes Bogtrykkeri, Copenhagen (1970).

56 ——, ROOTWELT, K., and HØRVEN, I. Cutaneous blood flow in cluster headache. *Headache*, **13**, 173–5 (1974).

57 —— and SJAASTAD, Ø. V. Histamine metabolism in cluster headache and migraine. *J. Neurol.*, **216**, 105–17 (1977).

58 SOMMERVILLE, B. W. The role of estradiol withdrawal in the etiology of menstrual migraine. *Neurology*, **22**, 355–65 (1972).

59 SPIRA, P. J., MYLECHARNE, E. J., and LANCE, J. W. The effects of humoral agents and antimigraine drugs on the cranial circulation of the monkey. *Res. clin. Stud. Headache*, **4**, 37 (1976).
60 STOWELL, A. Physiologic mechanisms and treatment of histamine in petrosal neuralgia. *Headache*, **9**, 187–94 (1970).
61 SYMONDS, C. A particular variety of headache. *Brain*, **79**, 217–32 (1956).
62 WALSH, J. P. and O'DOHERTY, D. S. A possible explanation of the mechanism of ophthalmoplegic migraine. *Neurology*, **10**, 1079 (1960).
63 WERNER, S. C. Clinical syndromes associated with gonadal failure in men. *Amer. J. Med.*, **3**, 52–66 (1947).

8 The management of cluster headache

The important principles concerning the successful treatment of cluster headache extend beyond the selection of proper drugs. In the post-examination conference, patients should be instructed in the current medical knowledge of cluster headache. This affords a better doctor–patient relationship, alleviates the patient's anxiety regarding serious complications, dispels misinformation, and allows him to participate in his treatment programme with greater awareness. Patient cooperation is a prerequisite to successful management.

Not all patients respond to first-line selection of medications. Follow-up visits are necessary to re-evaluate progress and to change medications, where indicated. Hence, patients are instructed to keep accurate records of their attacks which are to be presented every two to three weeks for the duration of the cluster period. Telephone communication is encouraged between visits if progress is not satisfactory.

The selection of particular drugs depend on compatability with other medications, history of untoward reaction or poor responsiveness, and the health of the patient. Drug selection will also depend on cluster headache type, frequency, timing of attacks, and the patient's age.

Avoidance

In all cases, patients are instructed to avoid afternoon naps and alcoholic beverages, including wine or beer. As noted in earlier chapters, alcohol will, in most instances, induce acute attacks during an active period; but not during remissions. Dietary influences, with the exception of alcohol, appear to have little importance in cluster headache.

Short sleep periods during the afternoon or early evening may induce acute cluster attacks. It may awaken the patient or begin soon after he awakens. Dexter[7] reports that cluster attacks, occurring during sleep, are likely to be associated with the REM state. It is possible that during naps, the latency of the REM periods are shorter.

Since light glare seems to be poorly tolerated during active periods, patients are advised to wear sunglasses and to avoid facing outside windows when seated indoors.

Bursts of anger, prolonged anticipation, excitement, and excessive physical activity are to be avoided, since in the relaxation period that follows, cluster attacks are apt to occur. We have also observed that prolonged or sustained periods (two weeks or more) of anger, 'hurt', rage, or frustration, experienced during remission periods, are often associated with a cluster period onset.

Not infrequently, cluster periods begin after alterations in sleep–wake cycles. Vacation trips, work-shift changes, new occupations, post-surgical periods, completion of university studies, etc. are conditions commonly associated with the cluster period onset. Although there are many variables associated with such life-style changes, alterations of sleep–wake patterns, which often accompany these changes, may be the most significant.

As discussed in Chapter 6, alterations in sleep–wake cycles, as often occur with 'jet-lag', influence the circadian rhythm of cerebral-amine secretion, affecting autonomic nervous system function, vasomotor control, antinociception, and emotional responses.[32, 55] If indeed, this scheme is relevant to the pathogenesis of cluster headache, then re-establishment of sleep–wake cycles may modify the active cluster period. This approach is presently being studied.

Prophylactic medication

At the present time, several medications are available that will prevent attacks during active cluster periods. Each are discussed in the following section. Specific treatment regimens are presented in a subsequent section.

Ergotamine

Ergotamine is an alpha-adrenergic blocking agent; and depresses central vasomotor centres. It acts peripherally as a vasoconstrictor agent directly stimulating smooth muscle of peripheral and extra-cranial blood vessels.

Because of its vasoconstrictive properties, ergotamine has been successfully used in migraine for many years. Spira, Mylecharane, and Lance[53] have demonstrated its selective action on extracranial blood vessels in monkeys. Edmeads, Hachinski, and Norris,[8] having studied the effects of ergotamine on cerebral blood-flow in humans, found no significant changes.

Spira, Mylecharane, and Lance[53] reported that intravenous injection of the equivalent of 0·25 mg in a 70-kg man had a peak effect in two to eleven minutes; its vasoconstrictor effect was maintained during a two-hour period. Meier and Schreier[40] showed that the first phase of the elimination half-life of ergotamine was five to six hours. Harris[23] had reported that ergotamine was effective in alleviating cluster attacks. Subsequently, Symonds[54] and Horton[27] advocated its use as an effective symptomatic medication in this condition. The value of ergotamine prophylaxis was first reported by K. A. Ekbom[11] in 1947. He had successfully treated 13 of 16 patients, using oral ergotamine tartrate, 2 mg, 2 to 3 times a day.

In 1958, Friedman and Mikropolous[14] reported that symptomatic treatment with ergotamine resulted in an 85 per cent success rate in 30 patients with cluster headache.

In our own series, of the first 100 patients treated, 79 per cent had obtained significant relief from sublingual or inhalant ergotamine preparations. It is well to remember that once the attack is in progress, the absorption of oral preparations is delayed, since gastric stasis may result in the presence of pain. Hence, this route of administration is not recommended for symptomatic treatment of acute cluster attacks. Although intravenous or intramuscular injections of ergotamine are the most effective routes of administration, their value is limited by inconvenience. Therefore, considering effectiveness and convenience, sublingual and inhalant medications remain preparations of choice (Table 8.1).

Side-effects and contraindications. Nausea and paresthesias of the extremities are commonly experienced following intramuscular or intravenous administration of ergotamine. Muscle pains, leg weakness, tachycardia, or bradycardia are less commonly reported. Side-effects, such as, nausea, vomiting and paresthesias occur more frequently with injectable ergotamine tartrate than with dihydroergotamine (DHE-45). All side-effects are less commonly experienced following oral, sublingual, or inhalation preparations.

Ergotamine should not be used in the presence of infection, particularly where the liver or kidneys are involved. Its use is contraindicated in peripheral vascular or coronary artery disease, hypertension, and pregnancy.

Table 8.1   Ergotamine preparations, strength and recommended dosage for symptomatic and prophylactic treatment of cluster headache

Preparations	Strength	Recommended Dosage
Symptomatic treatment		
Injectable		
Ergotamine tartrate		
(Gynergan)	1·0 mg	0·5 mg, i.m.
Dihydroergotamine		
(DHE-45)	1·0 mg	1·0 mg, i.m.
Suppository		
Ergotamine tartrate		
(Cafergot, Cafergot PB)	2·0 mg	One suppository
Sublingual		
Ergotamine tartrate		
(Ergomar, Ergostat)	2·0 mg	2·0 mg, sublingual. Repeat once in 30 min if necessary
Inhalation		
Ergotamine		
(Medihaler ergotamine)	0·36 mg	Three inhalations, 5 min apart if necessary
Prophylactic treatment		
Tablets		
Ergotamine tartrate		
(Cafergot, Cafergot PB, Wigraine)	1·0 mg	Tab 2, h.s. or Tab 1, b.i.d.–t.i.d.

It is of some interest that in two cases treated at our clinic, hallucinations were reported following the use of oral ergotamine preparations. Both patients had used LSD regularly several years earlier. The relative structural similarity of ergotamine to the hallucinogen may explain this untoward reaction.

Methysergide

Methysergide maleate (Sansert) is an ergot derivative (1-methyl-D-lysergic acid butanolamide), having potent antiserotonin effects. It potentiates the vasoconstrictive effects of norepinephrine on the external carotid artery system in man,[4] dogs,[47] and monkeys.[42] In the internal carotid artery, it antagonizes serotonin-induced constriction by both competitive and non-competitive mechanisms.[36] Its elimination half-life is approximately three hours.[40] As noted by Lovshin,[37] Sicuteri[50] reported the first study on the efficacy of methysergide prophylaxis in migraine and had included two cases of cluster headache. In the following year, four other studies were reported.[25,12,19,2] The largest of these series[19] included only 16 patients with cluster headache. Between 1961 and 1963, four additional reports were published.[13,22,21,50] Lovshin,[37] in 1963, reported good to excellent results in 110 out of 159 patients with cluster headache (69 per cent). This compared to a 77 per cent success rate averaged for all previous studies. Our own survey, reported in 1978, included 77 patients. Good to excellent results were found in 65 per cent[33] (Table 8.2). Although it would appear that the effectiveness of methysergide prophylaxis in cluster headache is less dramatic than reported earlier, it remains effective in approximately 70 per cent of cases.

Table 8.2   Results of methysergide maintenance therapy in cluster headache

Author(s)	Year	No. patients	Good to excellent results N (per cent)
Sicuteri[50]	1959	2	2 (100)
Heyck[25]	1960	8	8 (100)
Friedman[12]	1960	3	2 (67)
Graham[19]	1960	20	16 (80)
Bergouignan and Seilhean[2]	1960	3	3 (100)
Friedman and Losin[13]	1961	21	15 (71)
Harris[22]	1961	5	5 (100)
Hale and Reed[21]	1962	8	3 (38)
Lovshin[37]	1963	159	110 (69)
Kudrow[33]	1978	77	50 (65)

Methysergide has little value in the symptomatic treatment of cluster headache. Furthermore, prophylactic benefits appear to be limited to the episodic type. In 1978, we found that 41 out of 77 episodic patients had obtained better than 75 per cent improvement, and 9 out of 77 were partially improved, having obtained a 50–75 per cent benefit. In contrast, of 15 patients with chronic cluster, one improved markedly, two were partially benefited, and twelve (80 per cent) were considered failures.[33] Hence, methysergide is not recommended as a first-line prophylactic medication for chronic cluster headache. Furthermore, daily use for prolonged periods, as required in chronic cases, may lead to fibrotic complications.

Another limitation of methysergide is its loss of effectiveness in subsequent cluster periods, in the same individual. In an unpublished survey of 60 patients treated successfully with methysergide, we found that 20 per cent had become unresponsive to this agent when treated for a subsequent cluster period. Of 20 patients treated for a third cluster period, 40 per cent achieved poor results. This peculiar form of tolerance was first described by Lovshin.[37] He found that of 13 patients who had obtained excellent results when initially treated with methysergide, four (30 per cent) achieved less than excellent results during the second period. In three patients treated for a third period, only one continued to have excellent results.[37]

Side-effects and contraindications associated with methysergide therapy further limit the use of this drug. However, Lovshin[37] reported that in only 3 of 159 cluster patients (2 per cent) receiving methysergide, medication had to be discontinued, because of vomiting. An additional 19 patients experienced transient side-effects which abated with continued use. The most common side-effect was nausea.

In their report on methysergide prophylaxis in a mixed vascular (migraine and cluster) headache population, Friedman and Losin[13] listed the most common side-effects, in order of frequency: light-headedness, nausea, epigastric distress, and difficulty in concentration. In our own cluster population, the most frequently observed side-effects are: chest and leg muscle pains, nausea, paresthesias, light-headedness, cold extremities, and pedal oedema.

Peripheral vascular, cardiovascular, or fibrotic complications may result from chronic methysergide use. Nevertheless, intrinsic vasoconstriction of blood vessels may occur at any stage of treatment. In their series, Friedman and Losin[13] reported that one patient had complained of pain in both feet, numbness, and generalized muscle cramps, after only five days of methysergide therapy. Pulses were unobtainable on examination up to the level of the femoral pulse.[13]

In 1965, Graham[18] and Graham and Parnes[20] reported complications of retroperitoneal and endocardial fibrosis resulting from prolonged, non-interrupted methysergide therapy. Subsequently, Graham[16] reported 13 cases of pleuropulmonary fibrosis. He stated that although a half million patients had been treated with methysergide, fibrotic complications had been reported in only 100 cases. Where endocardial fibrosis had occurred he observed that the mitral valve lesions were similar to those of carcinoid heart disease; thus, he suggested a possible role of serotonin in the pathogenesis of methysergide fibrosis.[16]

Thus far, these complications have not been reported where methysergide had been used for no longer than three-month periods. On the basis of this observation, chronic methysergide treatment should be interrupted every three months, for one-month intervals.

BC-105

BC-105 is an anti-serotonin, antihistaminic agent, 4-(1-, methyl-4-piperidylidene)-9, 10-dihydro-4H-benzo{4,5}cyclo hepta {1,2-}thiophene. It was studied for prophylactic efficacy in migraine by Sicuteri, Franchi, and Del Bianco.[51] They reported that its prophylactic benefit in seven cluster patients was less satisfactory than that obtained in migraine patients. Ekbom[10] in 1969, published results of a controlled trial of BC-105 prophylaxis in 28 cases of episodic cluster headache. He found that 57 per cent of patients had obtained good to excellent results. Comparing results of BC-105 to those of ergotamine prophylaxis in ten cases, he found that BC-105 was superior in six; ergotamine was superior in two; and there was no difference in two cases.

Side-effects and complications. Of 23 cases, Ekbom[10] reported side-effects of drowsiness in ten (43·5 per cent), weight gain greater than two kilograms in eight (34·8 per cent), nausea in one, and anxiety in another case. Thus far, there have been no reported cases of fibrotic complications resulting from prophylactic treatment with BC-105.

Steroids

Horton[27] administered serial injections of ACTH to augment the response to histaminic desensitization. Horton[27] and Friedman and Mikropoulos[14] reported that cortisone alone, had little value.

MacNeal[38] found that the addition of triamcinalone to ergotamine prophylaxis offered significant benefit. Graham[17] had also recommended prednisone prophylaxis, for a four- to six-week period, as a viable alternative treatment of this disorder.

The first controlled study of prednisone prophylaxis in cluster headache was reported by Jammes[31] in 1975. He found that of 19 cluster patients resistant to methysergide or ergotamine therapy, 17 had obtained sustained relief following a single dose (30 mg) of prednisone. Subjects receiving placebo had a significantly greater attack frequency.

In our series of 77 episodic cluster patients who were unresponsive to methysergide, prednisone therapy resulted in marked relief in 76·6 per cent, partial improvement in 11·7 per cent, and no significant improvement in 11·7 per cent.

Of 15 chronic patients, 40 per cent had obtained marked improvement, and 33 per cent partial improvement. In recent years, prednisone has become the prophylactic medication of choice in episodic cluster headache; yet its action in this condition remains unknown.

The prednisone treatment regimen used at the California Medical Clinic for Headache is as follows: 40 mg per day for the first five days; 30 mg for five days; 20 mg for four days; 15 mg for three days; 10 mg for two days; and 5 mg for two days. The medication is taken in divided daily doses for an over-all period of three weeks. Where necessary, a second series may be prescribed following a one-week interval. At times, it is necessary to add ergotamine (2 mg h.s.) to the prednisone regimen, particularly when the dosage has been reduced to 15 mg per day (Table 8.3).

Table 8.3   Recommended schedule of prednisone prophylaxis

Dosage	Days
10 mg q.i.d.	5
10 mg t.i.d.	5
10 mg b.i.d.	4
5 mg t.i.d.	3
5 mg b.i.d.	2
5 mg daily	2

Side-effects and contraindications. In our clinic population, side-effects from prednisone occurred in the following order of frequency: insomnia (8 per cent); fluid retention (6 per cent); mood changes (5 per cent); and unexplained abdominal pain (2 per cent). Steroids should not be used in the presence of hypertension, diabetes, infection, peptic ulcer disease, or in association with immunization procedures. Its use is further contraindicated in the presence of diverticulosis. Regarding the latter disorder, we have seen two cases in which perforation of diverticula had occurred during short-term prednisone treatment for cluster headache. Neither patient had experienced symptoms of diverticulitis prior to treatment. In one, perforation occurred on the second day, by which time, the patient had received a total of 90 mg of prednisone. Palmer, Mason, and Adams[43] reported two cases of diverticula perforation on the fourth day of ACTH administration in one patient, and after two years of oral cortisone therapy, in the other. (These patients were being treated for conditions other than cluster headache.)

Lithium

Cyclic affective disorders have been shown to respond to lithium therapy. Since cluster headache occurs cyclically, Ekbom[9] investigated the possible benefit of lithium in this disorder. He treated five patients for up to 18 months; three patients had chronic, and two, episodic cluster headache. The chronic patients responded dramatically to lithium therapy, and subsequent withdrawal of medication resulted in exacerbation of attacks. Readministration caused significant relief. Although favourable, the results were not as beneficial in the episodic group as in the chronic cluster patients.

Encouraged by Ekbom's results,[9] we evaluated the efficacy of lithium in 32 patients, over a 32-week period.[34] All patients were diagnosed as having chronic cluster headache, and were resistant to, or intolerant of, methysergide, prednisone, and ergotamine. Patients had been advised to maintain their usual salt intake, refrain from use of all other drugs, and to report untoward effects. They were instructed to record their headaches daily, by rated severity (1 = mild, 2 = moderate, 3 = severe). A weekly index (HAI) was derived by multiplying the attack frequency by the severity. In addition, a headache index ratio (HAR) was calculated. This defines quantitative improvement by dividing 'lithium treatment HAI' by the 'pre-treatment HAI'. The percentage improvement is the reciprocal number of the HAR multiplied by 100. Lithium carbonate, 300–600 mg per day was used during the first week, increasing to 600–900 mg by the fourth week. The maintenance dose depended on the clinical response and severity of side effects, rather than serum lithium levels. The dose of lithium was reduced if serum levels were above 1·2 meq/l. Serum lithium levels were measured weekly for a month, and monthly thereafter.

Of 28 patients completing the study, 11 (42 per cent) obtained improvement ranging between 60 and 90 per cent. Fourteen (54 per cent) obtained a greater than 90 per cent improvement. Only one patient was considered unimproved. There appeared to be no difference in response between primary and secondary cluster headache-types (Table 8.4).

Table 8.4   Results of lithium treatment of 26 patients with chronic cluster headache

Cluster types	N	Mean age	Improvement (per cent)†					
			< 60		60–90		> 90	
			N	per cent	N	per cent	N	per cent
Primary	17	35	1	(6)	6	(38)	9	(56)
Secondary	11	41	0		5	(50)	5	(50)
Total or average	28	38	1	(4)	11	(42)	14	(54)

†Derived from headache index ratios.

The results of our study showed that lithium carbonate prophylaxis was beneficial in chronic cluster headache. Moderately long-term therapy did not lead to lithium intolerance. In fact, lower maintenance doses provided continued improvement after the twelfth week. Patients who had improved on lithium often experienced dramatic relief within the first week, which continued for the duration of the study (Fig. 8.1). They experienced, however, a 'run' of daily, mild cluster attacks for three or four consecutive days, every three to six weeks. Fewer still, developed occasional moderate to severe cluster attacks without having altered the maintenance dose. Because of the high incidence of alcohol use in a cluster population, it was not surprising that some patients continued to drink in spite of warnings. These patients noted that lithium had not prevented alcohol-induced cluster attacks. This suggests that although lithium may suppress central mechanisms responsible for spontaneous cluster attacks, it does not interfere with mechanisms of peripheral induction, as seen with alcohol.

Mathew[39] evaluated the response to lithium in 31 patients with cluster headache, of whom 14 were episodic, and 17 chronic. Lithium was found to be equally effective in both cluster types. Fifty-five per cent of all patients had obtained more than 90 per cent improvement; ten per cent, between 60 and 90 per cent; fifteen per cent, 25–60 per cent; and twenty per cent showed no improvement.

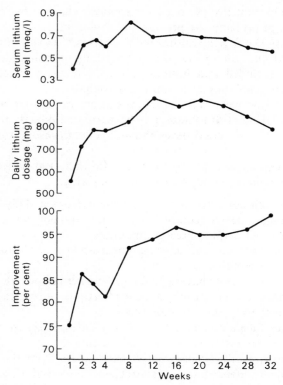

FIG. 8.1 Weekly improvements corresponding to lithium level and dosage. Represented are mean values for 28 chronic cluster patients. [From L. Kudrow.[34]]

Savoldi, Nappi, and Bono[46] reported that all of 12 cluster patients (10 chronic and 2 episodic) had obtained significant improvement during 2 to 18 months of treatment.

There is little doubt that lithium is effective in cluster headache; and it is probably the most effective of all prophylactic agents in chronic cluster. The action, however, by which it exerts its beneficial effects, remains unknown. Schou[49] has suggested that a feature common to all disorders responding to lithium therapy, is a cyclic, periodic, or episodic pattern. Not all episodic disorders are responsive to lithium, however.

Horrobin, Mtabaji, Manku, and Karmazyn[26] suggested that

lithium may influence peripheral vasomotor changes by inhibiting the effects of prolactin on prostaglandin biosynthesis.

Mellerup, Dam, Wildschidtz, and Rafaelsen,[41] having studied the effect of lithium on various diurnal rhythms on manic depressive patients, concluded that lithium may have a direct effect on the temperature-regulating centre in the hypothalamus.

In view of the cyclic and vasomotor character of cluster headache, the beneficial effect of lithium may be attributed directly to central regulation of cyclic biosynthesis and indirectly, to vasomotor regulation.

In our experience, having treated more than 100 patients with lithium carbonate, we have found the following:

1. Most lithium responders will benefit from a daily dose of 600 mg; some will require 900 mg a day, and only an occasional patient will require greater amounts.
2. Chronic patients appear to be more responsive to lithium, than those with episodic patterns.
3. Episodic patients having prolonged cluster periods, or who are resistant to other prophylactic medications, appear to respond better than typical episodic types.
4. Successful maintenance doses of only 300 mg a day are observed in approximately 10 per cent of patients.
5. Approximately 60 per cent of responders from the chronic group experience bursts of short cluster periods during uninterrupted lithium maintenance. Attacks, however, are generally less severe and of shorter duration.
6. Following cessation of lithium maintenance, approximately 20 per cent of chronic cluster responders become episodic.
7. Approximately 40 per cent of all cluster patients maintained on lithium require concomitant ergotamine prophylaxis for complete relief of headache.

Side-effects and complications. In our series of 32 patients, 4 were discontinued from further study because of severe side-effects resulting from lithium therapy; 3 had experienced recurrent, moderately severe, throbbing occipital pain, lasting from six to twelve hours in duration. One patient had experienced anorexia, vague abdominal discomfort, persistent nausea and vomiting, and rapid weight loss, all of which were relieved after lithium was discontinued.

Eight patients had experienced transient, mild to moderate side-effects. All, however, completed the study. Five out of eight exhibited tremor, especially during excitement of exertion. Four out of eight had episodes of mental confusion, decreased concentration and memory deficiency. Decreasing the lithium dosage eliminated these symptoms (Table 8.5). Otherwise, no relationship was found between lithium levels and adverse symptoms. This observation had also been reported by Schou[48] in patients treated for affective disorders.

Table 8.5 Frequency and description of side-effects during lithium therapy in 32 patients with chronic cluster headache

Severity of side-effects	N	(per cent)	Description	N
Severe—requiring discontinuation	4 ·	(12·5)	'Lithium headache'	3
			Abdominal pain and vomiting	1
Mild—allowing continuation	8	(25)	Tremor	5
			Thought dysfunction	4
			Lethargy	3
			Diarrhoea	3
			Insomnia	2
			Lightheadedness	2

The lithium ion is not metabolized, and approximately 80 per cent of the glomerula filtrate is reabsorbed along with sodium and water in the proximal tubule. In the presence of sodium deficiency, lithium reabsorption increases along with a compensatory increase in sodium reabsorption from the same site.[24] Since there is an inverse relationship between serum sodium levels and lithium reabsorption, then lithium should be used cautiously, if at all, in the presence of chronic diuretic therapy, or in cases requiring low salt diets.

Hypothyroidism, especially in women, may result during prolonged lithium therapy.[15] This is thought to result from impairment of iodotyrosine coupling and TSH blockade.[30]

Lithium may also produce a reversible nephrogenic diabetes insipitus, characterized by polyuria and polydipsia.[30]

Comparative success rates of methysergide, prednisone, and lithium prophylaxis

In 1977 we evaluated 92 patients with cluster headache for comparative responses to prophylactic treatment with methysergide, prednisone, and lithium carbonate;[33] 77 had episodic, and 15 chronic cluster. In all cases, the first course of treatment was methysergide,

8 mg a day in divided doses, for 21 days. Failure to respond favourably after ten days of treatment prompted the second course of medication, prednisone; 40 mg a day in divided doses, gradually tapered off over a period of 21 days. In cases of chronic cluster headache, failure to respond to prednisone signaled the onset of lithium therapy; lithium carbonate, 600 mg a day in two divided doses, for 7 days, and increased to 900 mg a day for an additional two weeks. Percentage of improvement for each patient was calculated by comparing pre-treatment and post-treatment headache indices. Improvement was divided into three grades: 0–47 per cent, considered failure; 50–74 per cent, partial improvement; and 75–100 per cent, marked improvement.

Table 8.6   Responses of 77 episodic cluster patients to methysergide and prednisone prophylaxis

Medication	Improvement					
	Partial		Marked		Over-all	
	N	(per cent)	N	(per cent)	N	(per cent)
Methysergide	9	(11·7)	41	(53·2)	50	(64·9)
Prednisone	9	(11·7)	59	(76·6)	68	(88·3)

Table 8.7   Responses of 15 chronic cluster patients to methysergide, prednisone, and lithium prophylaxis

Medication	Improvement					
	Partial		Marked		Over-all	
	N	(per cent)	N	(per cent)	N	(per cent)
Methysergide	2	(13·3)	1	(6·7)	3	(20·0)
Prednisone	5	(33·3)	6	(40·0)	11	(73·3)
Lithium	0	(0)	13	(86·7)	13	(86·7)

Results are summarized in Tables 8.6 and 8.7. Prednisone was found to be significantly better than methysergide in either episodic ($p < 0.05$) or chronic ($p < 0.001$) cluster groups. Lithium administered to chronic cluster patients solely, was significantly superior to methysergide ($p < 0.001$). In chronic cluster, the over-all response to prednisone was less than that of lithium, but the difference was not significant. Fifty per cent improvement or more, was found in only 20 per cent of patients treated with methysergide; however 73·3 and 86·7 per cent improved, following treatment with prednisone and lithium, respectively.

Other medications

Indomethacin (Indocin) is a non-steroidal drug having anti-inflammatory, anti-pyretic, and analgesic properties.

In 1976, Sjaastad and Dale[52] reported that the administration of indomethacin to patients with chronic paroxysmal hemicrania (CPH) resulted in dramatic remissions. CPH is a variant of chronic cluster headache. Furthermore, occasional patients with chronic cluster headache, other than CPH, obtain relief. Therefore, in cases unresponsive to other prophylactic medication, a trial of indomethacin therapy is indicated. The dosage schedule is 25 mg, three times a day, eventually decreased to the lowest effective maintenance dosage.

Side-effects and complications. The most common side effect of this medication is gastrointestinal. Indomethacin should be used with caution in patients having a history of peptic ulcer, epilepsy, Parkinsonism, and psychiatric disorders. Although rare, corneal deposits and retinal complications resulting from prolonged therapy have been reported.

Cyproheptadine (Periactin) is an antihistamine and serotonin antagonist, similar in structure and action to BC-105. Although commonly used in the United States for various conditions, its efficacy in the prophylactic treatment of cluster headache has not been proved. In our experience, therapeutic doses of cyproheptadine cause profound tiredness in most patients, precluding its use.

Symptomatic treatment of cluster attacks

Ergotamine

As stated earlier in this chapter, ergotamine is effective in approximately 80 per cent of all cases. Not all attacks, however, are successfully treated in a given patient. Ergotamine is less effective if used too late in an attack, and is sometimes ineffective for some attacks, without apparent explanation; occasional attacks are entirely unresponsive, even when medication is properly used.

Oxygen inhalation

Oxygen inhalation is an effective method of aborting acute cluster attacks. It is similar to ergotamine in its effectiveness and has the additional advantage of having neither side-effects nor conditions which contraindicate its use; the only disadvantage is inconvenience.

Horton[27] was the first to recommend 100 per cent oxygen inhalation at the onset of acute cluster attacks, but in combination with DHE-45, intramuscularly. Friedman and Mikropoulos[14] reported on its favourable effects, but held that ergotamine appeared to be more effective. Graham[17] stated that occasional patients had obtained relief from breathing 100 per cent oxygen for 15 minutes.

We systematically evaluated the symptomatic response to oxygen inhalation in cluster headache. Fifty-five consecutive patients, returning for routine office visits, were selected for study. All were allowed to continue prophylactic medication regardless of its success rate, since only the response of attacks to oxygen inhalation was being studied, and not attack frequency.

At the commencement of the attack, patients were instructed to breathe oxygen from a loosely applied facial mask, at a rate of 7 l/min for a period of 15 minutes. A minimum of ten attacks were treated in this manner. Patients recorded the intensity (3, severe; 2, moderate; 1, dull), and duration of attacks, from the onset of oxygen inhalation. Successful response was based on two criteria; at least seven out of ten attacks were either aborted or reduced to a dull intensity, within 15 minutes of oxygen inhalation.

Oxygen tanks (244 cm³) and attached regulators were rented from one supplier and pretested before delivery to the subjects' homes.

Of 52 patients completing the study, 45 were men and 7, women. All of the women were diagnosed as having episodic cluster. Nineteen men had chronic and 26, episodic types. Mean ages were 48 years for males and 51 years for females.

In the episodic group, 80·8 per cent of males and 71·4 per cent of females were significantly benefited. Of the chronic males, 68·4 per cent achieved success. In all, 75 per cent of the patients obtained significant responses (Table 8.8).

In order to determine whether favourable responses were age related, a comparison was made of patients under 50 years of age to patients over 49 years of age. In the former group, 22 out of 26 patients (84·6 per cent) responded favourably. This was significantly

Table 8.8   Beneficial effects of oxygen inhalation on acute attacks in episodic and chronic cluster groups

Sex and type of cluster	N	Mean age	Benefited by oxygen†	
			N	(per cent)
Males				
Episodic	26	49·7	21	(80·8)
Chronic	19	45·9	13	(68·4)
Subtotal	45	48·1	34	(75·6)
Females				
Episodic	7	51·3	5	(71·4)
Chronic	0	0	0	(0)
Subtotal	7	51·3	5	(71·4)
Total	52	48·5	39	(75·0)

†Abort 70 per cent of all attacks within a 15-min period.

better than the response from the older group ($p < 0.05$), where 17 out of 26 patients (65·4 per cent) had achieved beneficial results. The best responders to symptomatic oxygen inhalation were *episodic* patients under 50 years of age; 13 out of 14 (92·9 per cent). Conversely, the worst responders were *chronic* patients over 49 years of age; four out of seven (57·1 per cent). The numbers were too small for statistical testing of significant differences (Table 8.9). Finally, 39 patients successfully aborted or reduced 293 attacks. Headache relief occurred 62 per cent of the time within the first seven minutes

Table 8.9   Results of oxygen inhalation on cluster attacks. Comparison of two age groups

Age groups	N	Improved	
		N	(per cent)
Under-50			
Episodic	14	13	(92·9)
Chronic	12	9	(75·0)
Total	26	22	(84·6)
Over 49			
Episodic	19	13	(68·4)
Chronic	7	4	(57·1)
Total	26	17	(65·4)

of oxygen inhalation; 31 per cent within eight to ten minutes; and 6·8 per cent, within 11 to 15 minutes.

It would appear from our results that oxygen is an effective symptomatic treatment modality for the cluster attack. Although oxygen inhalation had not been compared to ergotamine responses in this study, oxygen inhalation caused no side-effects, appears to be safer, and is not contraindicated by cardiovascular, peripheral vascular, pulmonary, hepatic, or renal disease.

Another favourable aspect of oxygen inhalation was the rapidity with which it afforded significant pain relief. These results are comparable to our experience with ergotamine sublingual or inhalator administrations.

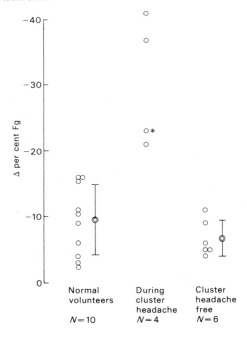

Fig. 8.2   To show mean hemispheric Fg changes during 100 per cent oxygen inhalation in 3 patients during cluster headache. There is a diffuse and excessive reduction of mean hemispheric Fg values which are more than three times that seen in normals. A fourth patient tested immediately (30 min) after the cluster headache had subsided, likewise shows an excessive vasoconstrictor response (*). An additional 6 patients with cluster headache were tested when they were free of headache (more than 12 hours after headache had subsided). All showed a normal vasoconstrictor response. [Reproduced with permission of F. Sakai & J. S. Meyer.[44]]

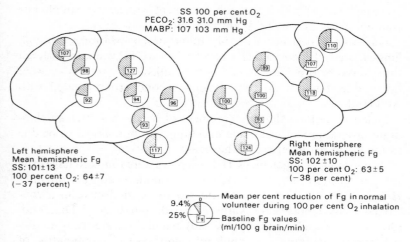

FIG. 8.3 To show serial measurements of Fg before and during 100 per cent oxygen inhalation in a 43-year-old man during cluster headache located behind the right eye. There is an excessive vasoconstrictor response noted diffusely throughout both hemispheres and the brain stem cerebellar regions. [Reproduced with permission of F. Sakai & J. S. Meyer.[44]]

The mechanism by which oxygen inhalation interrupts the cluster attack is unknown. Sakai and Meyer[45] had shown earlier that profound bihemispheric increases in cerebral blood-flow, particularly on the contralateral side, occurs consistently during the cluster attack. More recently, they have demonstrated that 100 per cent oxygen, administered during the attack, promptly reduced cerebral blood-flow and pain[44] (Figs. 8.2 and 8.3). They suggested that this hyper-reactivity of cerebral blood vessels to oxygen may be due to its potentiation of catecholamines, serotonin, and other vasoconstricting substances at the receptor level.

Other treatment modalities having questionable value

Medications

Histamine desensitization as first proposed by Horton, McLean, and Craig[29] was reported to shorten cluster periods in 95 per cent of their series. Other investigators, however, could not achieve this result, and expressed doubt about the validity of the procedure.[14, 35, 54]

Horton[28] had admitted that this treatment was neither simple nor commonplace, and was fraught with pitfalls.

Our own experience with histamine desensitization, although limited, was not encouraging. Indeed, when ACTH was administered three days before initiating histamine injections, responses were favourable, but not different from a second group treated with ACTH alone.

Dalessio[6] reports that improvement of headaches after an elaborate programme of histamine injections was not shown to be due to the desensitizing effect of this agent.

Antihistamines which block H-1 receptors were found to have little value in cluster headache by Horton,[29] Kunkle,[35] and Friedman.[14] H-2 receptor blockers were considered to be ineffective in a controlled study reported by Anthony, Lord, and Lance.[1] Diamond, Graham, and Kudrow (not published) in a multicentre study involving 60 patients, found no significant responses to a combination of H-1 (chlorpheniramine) of H-2 (cimetidine) receptor blocking agents.

Dimethyl sulphoxide (DSMO) is a substance which is rapidly absorbed through skin and is believed to have analgesic properties. Blumenthal and Fuchs[3] treated five cluster patients with this substance and found that only 25 per cent had reported good results.

Cryosurgery

In 1973, Cook[5] reported a 75 per cent success rate in the treatment of vascular headache using a cryosurgical technique. The superficial, temporal, and occipital arteries, as well as the sphenopalatine ganglion, were frozen at −160°C. Of 106 patients thus treated, 51 (48 per cent) had reported a 75 per cent improvement, ten of whom were 100 per cent relieved at the end of a six-month follow-up period.

With the full cooperation of Dr Cook and his patients, we undertook a two-year follow-up study to determine the efficacy of this procedure. Having reviewed all pertinent office charts, questionnaires were mailed to post-operative patients at eight-month intervals, for the two-year period. The questionnaires were designed to reaffirm the diagnosis of cluster headache, and to obtain pre- and post-operative headache frequency, severity, duration, and remission-length. As a means of sampling questionnaire's responses, eight patients were contacted directly by telephone, and two were personally interviewed.

Of 38 male patients diagnosed as having cluster headache, 14 were excluded because of non-compliance or other reasons. In the remaining 24 patients, 18 had episodic, and 6, chronic cluster headache. The mean ages were 47 and 49 years, respectively. The mean age of both groups was 47 years.

Of nine episodic patients having usual remission periods ranging between one and six months, 5 (55·5 per cent) remained headache-free at the end of the two-year follow-up period. In patients having pre-operative remission periods between 7–12 months or 13–18 months, no success was obtained. Only 27·8 per cent of all episodic patients remained headache-free for a two-year period following surgery.

Table 8.10 Sustained remissions, two years following cryosurgery in 24 cluster-headache males

Pre-op remission duration (months)	N	Mean age	Two years post-op remission	
			N	(per cent)
Episodic	1–18	18	47	5	(27·8)
	1–6	9	46	5	(55·6)
	7–12	7	47	0	
	13–18	2	60	0	
Chronic		6	49	2	(33·3)
Total or mean		24†	47	6	(25·0)

†Surgical complications: ipsilateral facial numbness in 33·3 per cent of cases.

Only two out of six patients (33·3 per cent) with chronic cluster headache had obtained a two-year post-operative remission. However, of the four chronic patients who had not obtained two-year remissions, two had been converted to an episodic state. Of all twenty-four patients having episodic and cluster headache, only six (25 per cent) were considered cryosurgical successes at the end of two years follow-up. It should also be noted that 33·3 per cent of all patients complained of sustained ipsilateral facial numbness following the surgery (Table 8.10).

It would appear that the greatest benefit of Dr Cook's cryosurgical procedure was obtained by patients who had a previous history of short or no remission periods. Although the study was limited to a two-year follow-up period, the benefit of this procedure in chronic cases is apparent, since two patients were completely relieved of their attacks for a two-year period, and another two had been converted to an episodic state.

Our results suggest that typical episodic patients having remission periods of seven months or more would benefit least from this procedure. Cryosurgery of the sphenopalatine ganglia may be a worthwhile procedure in chronic patients; or in episodic cases having shortened remission periods.

Other surgical procedures are discussed in Chapter 7.

Biofeedback training, psychiatry, hypnosis, physical therapy, and *manipulation techniques* appear to be of little value in either acute or prophylactic treatment of cluster headache. Although there have been no reported controlled studies that would validate or invalidate these procedures in cluster headache, impressions gained from experienced patients lead us to believe that such modalities have little value.

Selection of medications

Prophylactic regimens

Based on the experience of having treated approximately 500 cluster patients at the California Medical Clinic for Headache, we have established specific first-line treatment regimens according to the following criteria:

1. Previous response to prior prophylactic medications;
2. Adverse reactions to prior prophylactic medications;
3. Presence of disorders which contraindicate the use of specific medication;
4. Age of the patient;
5. Frequency of attacks.

Regarding the first three criteria, drugs which are either ineffective, non-tolerated, or contraindicated, are omitted from consideration. In cases where these conditions do not exist the choice of first-line agents depends on the patients' age and frequency of attacks.

It should be noted that the goal of adequate prophylaxis is not 100 per cent prevention of all attacks. Reduced frequency, severity, or duration of attacks, should be weighed against the hazards of over-medication. Furthermore, 100 per cent prevention is unnecessary since adequate symptomatic medication is available in the event

Table 8.11   Selection of prophylactic medication in episodic cluster headache according to age and attack frequency

Criteria	Prophylactic medication		
Age and attack frequency	First-line	Second-line‡	Third-line
One attack daily any age	Ergotamine 2 mg, p.o. two hours before expected attack	See 'two or more daily attacks'	
Two or more daily attacks			
Under 35	Methysergide 2 mg every 6–8 hours	Prednisone†	Ergotamine, 2 mg, p.o. every 12 hours
35–50	Prednisone†	Ergotamine 2 mg, p.o. every 12 hrs.	Lithium, 300 mg, b.i.d.-t.i.d., plus ergotamine, p.o., 1 mg, t.i.d. or 2 mg, h.s.
> 50	Lithium 300 mg (b.i.d.–t.i.d.)	Lithium, 300 mg (b.i.d.–t.i.d.) plus ergotamine, 1 mg p.o., t.i.d. or 2 mg, h.s.	Prednisone† (with close observation)

† For dose schedule, see Table 8.3.   ‡If first-line medication is unsuccessful.

of breakthrough attacks. Our treatment schedules are outlined in Table 8.11.

In episodic patients under 35 years of age, experiencing two or more daily attacks, methysergide (Sansert) is selected as the first-line medication. It should be taken every eight hours for the first five days, and increased to every six hours if the response is poor. Methysergide is usually effective in young people, and in those who had previously used it once or twice, or never at all. Resistance often occurs after prior treatment of several periods.

If methysergide proves ineffective it is tapered off over a period of two days, and prednisone prophylaxis is instituted, as outlined in Table 8.3. In the event that prednisone therapy is unsuccessful, or if after three weeks of therapy, attacks continue, then oral ergotamine (Cafergot, Wigraine) is prescribed; two tablets, every twelve hours.

Episodic cluster patients over 35 years of age are likely to be less responsive to methysergide than the younger population. Thus, when attacks occur with a frequency of two or more a day, in patients between the ages of 35 and 50, prednisone is recommended as the first-line prophylactic medication. Approximately 10 per cent of patients are unresponsive or intolerant to this medication, and in rare cases, attacks are exacerbated. In such an event, the steroid is rapidly tapered off and ergotamine prophylaxis is instituted and maintained. Lithium carbonate, 300 mg, used every 8 to 12 hours, may be added to the regimen if ergotamine alone is inadequate.

Populations over 50 years of age are generally more resitant to prophylactic efforts. Selection of medication is further complicated, in this age group, by a higher incidence of undetected or overt disorders, for example, coronary artery disease, recurrent peptic ulcer history, and diverticulosis. Therefore, it is more prudent to avoid drugs such as methysergide or prednisone, wherever possible.

The first-choice prophylactic medication in episodic patients over fifty years of age is lithium carbonate, 300 mg, every 8 to 12 hours. Initially, it should be taken every 12 hours, for a period of one week; and increased to every 8 hours, if ineffective in lower doses. The majority of patients responsive to lithium obtain significant and sometimes dramatic relief from 600 mg in divided, daily doses. In many patients higher amounts cause tremor although it is easily tolerated.

Serum lithium blood levels are obtained after one week, where the maintenance dosage is 900 mg a day, or more. Subsequent blood levels may be obtained after one month, and bimonthly thereafter. Blood levels are obtained every three months, in patients using 600 mg per day.

If results are unsatisfactory after two weeks of maximal treatment with lithium, ergotamine is added to the regimen, as indicated in Table 8.11. Prednisone is the third-line medication, but in this older age group, it should be used with caution.

Regardless of age, attacks that occur in the middle of sleep are most effectively treated with oral ergotamine (2 mg), at bedtime. It should be taken at least two hours before the expected attack.

Symptomatic treatment

As noted earlier, oxygen inhalation is effective and safe. Oxygen tanks and regulators may be rented from medical supply or other rental agencies. Tanks may be kept at home or at one's place of business for acute attacks. Oxygen inhalation is preferred to ergotamine preparations, where ergotamine is:

a. Being used prophylactically;
b. Causing side-effects;
c. Contraindicated or ineffective.

Unlike ergotamine, oxygen may be used repeatedly, without untoward effects.

Where ergotamine is preferred, sublingual or inhalant preparations are recommended. It should be used at the very onset of the attack. Sublingual preparations may be repeated only once or twice, after 15-minute intervals. Inhalants may be used three times, in 5-minute intervals, for a given attack. In general, ergotamine use should be limited to a maximum of 4 mg per 24-hour period.

Chronic cluster headache

Prednisone prophylaxis has limited value in chronic cluster headache since patients cannot be maintained on this medication for extended periods of time without increased hazard. In some cases, however, a three-week course of prednisone therapy may be valuable to 'break up' a bout of particularly frequent attacks.

Lithium carbonate is the most effective preventative medication in chronic cluster headache. Initial and maintenance doses and serum levels, as discussed earlier in episodic cluster, apply also to chronic patients. It is often necessary to supplement lithium maintenance with ergotamine. Although it has not been demonstrated under controlled conditions, the combination of the two drugs appear to have a potentiating effect. It is likely that this combination affects two or more pathways involved in cluster headache.

References

1 ANTHONY, M., LORD, G. D. A., and LANCE, J. W. Controlled trials of cimetidine in migraine and cluster headache. *Headache*, **18**, 261–4 (1978).
2 BERGOUIGNAN, M. and SEILHEAN, A. The place of anti-serotonins in the treatment of migraine and vasomotor headache. *Presse med.*, **68**, 2176–8 (1960).
3 BLUMENTHAL, L. S. and FUCHS, M. The clinical use of dimethyl sulfoxide on various headaches, musculoskeletal, and other general medical disorders. *Ann. NY Acad. Sci.*, **147**, 572–85 (1967).
4 CARROLL, P. R., EBELING, P. W., and GLOVER, W. E. The responses of

the human temporal and rabbit ear artery to 5-hydroxytryptamine and some of its antagonists. *Aust. J. exp. Biol. med. Sci.*, **52**, 813 (1974).

5 COOK, N. Cryosurgery of migraine. *Headache*, **12**, 143–50 (1973).

6 DALESSIO, D. J. *Wolff's headache and other head pain.* (3rd edn.), pp. 349–50. Oxford University Press, New York. (1972).

7 DEXTER, J. D. and RILEY, T. L. Studies in nocturnal migraine. *Headache*, **15**, 51–62 (1975).

8 EDMEADS, J., HACHINSKI, V. C., and NORRIS, J. W. Ergotamine and the cerebral circulation. *Hemicrania*, **7**, 6 (1976).

9 EKBOM, K. Litium vid kroniska symptom av cluster headache. Preliminärt Meddelande. *Pousc. Med.*, **19**, 148–56 (1974).

10 ——. Prophylactic treatment of cluster headache with a new serotonin antagonist, BC 105. *Acta Neurol. Scand.*, **45**, 601–10 (1969).

11 EKBOM, K. A. Ergotamine tartrate orally in Horton's 'histaminic cephalgia' (also called Harris's 'ciliary neuralgia'). A new method of treatment. *Acta Psychiat. Scand.* (*Suppl.*), **46**, 106–13 (1947).

12 FRIEDMAN, A. P. Clinical observations with 1-methyl-lysergic acid butanolamide (UML-491) in vascular headache. *Angiology*, **11**, 364–6 (1960).

13 —— and LOSIN, S. Evaluation of UML-491 in treatment of vascular headaches: an analysis of the effects of 1-methyl-d-lysergic acid (+) butanolamide bimaleate (methysergide). *Arch. Neurol.*, **4**, 241–5 (1961).

14 —— and MIKROPOULOS, H. E. Cluster headaches. *Neurology (Minneapolis)*, **8**, 63 (1958).

15 FYRÖ, B., PETTERSON, U. and SEDVALL, G. Time course for the effect of lithium on thyroid function in men and women. *Acta Psychiat. Scand.*, **49**, 230–8 (1973).

16 GRAHAM, J. R. Cardiac and pulmonary fibrosis during methysergide therapy for headaches. *Amer. J. med. Sci.*, **245**, 23–34 (1967).

17 ——. Cluster headache. In *Pathogenesis and treatment of headache* (ed. O. Appenzeller), pp. 93–108. Spectrum Publications, New York (1976).

18 ——. Possible renal complications of Sansert (methysergide) therapy for headache. *Headache*, **5**, 12–13 (1965).

19 ——. Use of a new compound, UML-491 (1-methyl-d-lysergic acid butanolamide), in the prevention of various types of headache: a pilot study. *New Engl. J. Med.*, **263**, 1273–7 (1960).

20 —— and PARNES, L. R. Possible cardiac and reno-vascular complications of Sansert therapy. *Headache*, **5**, 14–18 (1965).

21 HALE, A. F. and REED, A. F. Prophylaxis of frequent vascular headache with methysergide. *Amer. J. med. Sci.*, **243**, 92–152 (1962).

22 HARRIS, M. C. Prophylactic treatment of migraine headache and histamine cephalgia with a serotonin antagonist (methysergide). *Ann. Allergy*, **19**, 500–4 (1961).

23 HARRIS, W. Ciliary (migrainous) neuralgia and its treatment. *Brit. med. J.*, **1**, 457 (1936).

24 HEWICK, D. S. Patient factors influencing lithium dosage. In *Lithium in medical practice* (ed. F. N. Johnson and S. Johnson), pp. 355–63. University Park Press, Baltimore, Maryland (1978).

25 HEYCK, H. Serotonin antagonists in the therapy of migraine and Bing's erythroprosopalgia or Horton's syndrome. *Schweiz med. Wochenschr.*, **90**, 203–9 (1960).

26 HORROBIN, D. F., MTABAJI, J. P., MANKU, M. S., and KARMAZYN, M. Lithium as a regulator of hormone-stimulated prostaglandin synthesis. In *Lithium in medical practice* (ed. F. N. Johnson and S. Johnson), pp. 243–6. University Park Press, Baltimore, Maryland (1978).

27 HORTON, B. T. Histamine cephalgia. *Lancet*, **72**, 92 (1952).

28 ——. Histamine cephalgia: differential diagnosis and treatment: 1,176 patients 1937–1955. *Proc. Staff Meet. Mayo Clin.*, **31**, 325 (1956).

29 ——, MCLEAN, A. R., and CRAIG, W. MCK. The use of histamine in the treatment of specific types of headache. *Proc. Staff Meet. Mayo Clin.*, **14**, 257 (1939).

30 HULLIN, R. P. The place of lithium in biological psychiatry. In *Lithium in medical practice* (ed. F. N. Johnson and S. Johnson), pp. 433–54. University Park Press, Baltimore, Maryland (1978).

31 JAMMES, J. L. The treatment of cluster headache with prednisone. *Dis. nerv. Syst.* **36**, 375–6 (1975).

32 KLEIN, K. E., BRÜNER, H., HOLTMANN, H., REHME, H., STOLTZE, J., STEINHOFF, W. D., and WEGMANN, H. M. Circadian rhythm of pilots' efficiency and effects of multiple time zone travel. *Aerospace Med.*, **41**, 125–31 (1970).

33 KUDROW, L. Comparative results of prednisone, methysergide, and lithium therapy in cluster headache. In *Current concepts in migraine research* (ed. R. Greene), pp. 159–63. Raven Press, New York (1978).

34 ——. Lithium prophylaxis for chronic cluster headache. *Headache*, **17**, 15–18 (1977).

35 KUNKLE, E. C., PFEIFFER, J. B. JR., WILHOIT, W. M., and HAMRICK, L. W. JR. Recurrent brief headache in cluster pattern. *Trans. Amer. neurol. Assoc.*, **77**, 240 (1952) and *North Carolina med. J.*, **15**, 510 (1954).

36 LANCE, J. W. *Mechanisms and management of headache.* (3rd edn.) Butterworths, London (1978).

37 LOVSHIN, L. L. Treatment of histaminic cephalgia with methysergide (UML-491). *Dis. nerv. Syst.*, **24**, 3–7 (1963).

38 MACNEAL, P. S. Useful therapeutic approaches to the patient with 'problem headache'. *Headache*, **14**, 186–9 (1975).

39 MATHEW, N. T. Clinical subtypes of cluster headache and response to lithium therapy. *Headache*, **18**, 26–30 (1978).

40 MEIER, J. and SCHREIER, E. Human plasma levels of some antimigraine drugs. *Headache*, **16**, 96 (1976).

41 MELLERUP, E. T., DAM, H., WILDSCHIDTZ, G., and RAFAELSEN, O. J. Lithium effect on various diurnal rhythms in manic, melancholic patients. In *Lithium in medical practice* (ed. F. N. Johnson and S. Johnson), pp. 267–70. University Park Press, Baltimore, Maryland (1978).

42 MYLECHARANE, E. J., SPIRA, P. J., MISBACH, J., DUCKWORTH, J. W., and LANCE, J. W. Effects of methysergide, pizotifen, and ergotamine in the monkey cranial circulation. *Eur. J. Pharmacol.* (In press).

43 PALMER, T. H. JR., MASON, P. J. H., and ADAMS, A. L. Diverticulitis

of the colon with perforation during cortisone and ACTH therapy. *J. Maine med. Assoc.*, **150**, 349–51 (1955).

44 SAKAI, F., and MEYER, J. S. Abnormal cerebrovascular reactivity in patients with migraine and cluster headache. *Headache*, **19**, 257–66 (1979).

45 —— and ——. Regional cerebral hemodynamics during migraine and cluster headaches measured by the ^{133}Xe inhalation method. *Headache*, **18**, 122–32 (1978).

46 SAVOLDI, F., NAPPI, G., and BONO, G. Lithium salts in treatment of idiopathic headaches and of facial pain syndromes. In *Proceedings of the Polish–Italian Meeting of Neurology*, Varenna, June 1978 (ed. P. Pinelli).

47 SAXENA, P. R. The effect of antimigraine drugs on the vascular responses of 5-hydroxytryptamine and related biogenic substances on the external carotid bed of dogs: possible pharmacological implications to their antimigraine action. *Headache*, **12**, 44 (1972).

48 SCHOU, M. Lithium in psychiatric therapy and prophylaxis. *J. psychiat. Res.*, **6**, 67–95 (1968).

49 ——. The range of clinical uses of lithium. In *Lithium in medical practice* (ed. F. N. Johnson and S. Johnson), pp. 21–39. University Park Press, Baltimore, Maryland (1978).

50 SICUTERI, F. Prophylactic and therapeutic properties of 1-methyl-lysergic acid butanolamide in migraine: preliminary report. *Int. Arch. Allergy appl. Immunol.*, **15**, 300–7 (1959).

51 ——, FRANCHI, G., and DEL BIANCO, P. L. An antaminic drug BC 105, in the prophylaxis of migraine. *Int. Arch. Allergy*, **31**, 78–93 (1967).

52 SJAASTAD, O. and DALE, I. A new (?) clinical headache entity 'Chronic Paroxysmal Hemicrania' 2. *Acta Neurol. Stand.*, **54**, 140–59 (1976).

53 SPIRA, P. J., MYLECHARANE, E. J., and LANCE, J. W. The effects of humoral agents and antimigraine drugs on the cranial circulation of the monkey. *Res. clin. Stud. Headache*, **4**, 37 (1976).

54 SYMONDS, C. A particular variety of headache. *Brain*, **79**, 217 (1956).

55 WEITZMAN, E. D., KRIPKE, D. F., GOLDMACHER, D., McGREGOR, P., and NOGEIRE, C. Acute reversal of the sleep–waking cycle in man. *Arch. Neurol.*, **22**, 483–9 (1970).

Index